# CULTURE
and
# HEALTH

# WILEY SERIES

in

# CULTURE AND PROFESSIONAL PRACTICE

*Editor*

**Daphne Keats**

*The University of Newcastle, Australia*

*Culture and the Child:*
*A Guide for Professionals in Child Care and Development*
Daphne Keats

*Communication and Culture:*
*A Guide for Practice*
Cynthia Gallois
and
Victor J. Callan

*Culture and Health*
Malcolm MacLachlan

Further titles in preparation

*Cultural Influences on Education and Schooling*

*Culture and the Law*

# CULTURE
## and
# HEALTH

## Malcolm MacLachlan
*Trinity College, Dublin, Ireland*

## JOHN WILEY & SONS

Chichester · New York · Weinheim · Brisbane · Singapore · Toronto

Copyright © 1997 by John Wiley & Sons Ltd,
Baffins Lane, Chichester,
1UD, England

79777
1243 779777
and customer service enquiries):
).uk
ge on http://www.wiley.co.uk
or http://www.wiley.com

k may be reproduced, stored in a retrieval
y any means, electronic, mechanical,
herwise, except under the terms of the
Copyright, Designs and Patents Act 1988 or under the terms of a licence issued by
the Copyright Licensing Agency, 90 Tottenham Court Road, London, UK W1P 9HE,
without the permission in writing of the Publisher.

*Other Wiley Editorial Offices*

John Wiley & Sons, Inc., 605 Third Avenue,
New York, NY 10158-0012, USA

VCH Verlagsgesellschaft mbH, Pappelallee 3,
D-69469 Weinheim, Germany

Jacaranda Wiley Ltd, 33 Park Road, Milton,
Queensland 4064, Australia

John Wiley & Sons (Asia) Pte Ltd, 2 Clementi Loop #02-01,
Jin Xing Distripark, Singapore 129809

John Wiley & Sons (Canada) Ltd, 22 Worcester Road,
Rexdale, Ontario M9W 1L1, Canada

*Library of Congress Cataloging-in-Publication Data*
MacLachlan, Malcolm.
    Culture and health : psychological perspectives on problems and
 practice / Malcolm MacLachlan.
        p.    cm. — (Wiley series in culture and professional practice)
    Includes bibliographical references and index.
    ISBN 0-471-96626-6 (pbk.)
    1. Transcultural medical care. 2. Ethnic groups—Health and
hygiene. 3. Minorities—Health and hygiene. I. Title.
II. Series.
RA418.5.T73M33    1997
362.1—dc21                                             97-8648
                                                          CIP

*British Library Cataloguing in Publication Data*

A catalogue record for this book is available from the British Library

ISBN 0-471-96626-6

Typeset in 11/13pt Palatino by Dorwyn Ltd, Rowlands Castle, Hants
Printed and bound in Great Britain by Bookcraft (Bath) Ltd, Midsomer Norton,
Somerset
This book is printed on acid-free paper responsibly manufactured from sustainable
forestation, for which at least two trees are planted for each one used for paper
production.

*To my parents:*
*for the fun*
*of life*

# CONTENTS

# ABOUT THE AUTHOR

*Mac MacLachlan* trained as a clinical psychologist at the Institute of Psychiatry, University of London, and has worked as a clinician, consultant in health service development and university lecturer in both Europe and Africa. He is the Director of the recently established Health Psychology Unit at Trinity College, Dublin, and specializes in researching the interplay between culture and health, and in implementing intervention programmes to promote health.

# SERIES PREFACE

The Wiley Series in Culture and Professional Practice provides a guide for professionals whose daily work in a number of fields requires them to consider the role of cultural factors in the needs and behaviour of their clients.

Whether through immigration, urbanisation, the aftermath of wars and natural disasters, the movement of people around the world in the large multinational business organisations, or even the world-wide development of tourist travel, few are untouched by contact with people of cultures different from their own. Professional help is often called for, but too often professional training courses do not give much consideration to cultural issues. The volumes in this Series will offer some practical help for these situations.

The Series covers some of the most frequent professional situations in which culture is an important influence.

I. *Culture and the Child* deals with issues in child care and development. Topics include temperamental and behavioural differences, the family, social interactions, children's motivations and anxieties and dealing with children in multicultural social contexts.

II. *Culture and Communication* deals with problems of communicating in business and interactions in many different settings.

III. *Culture and Health* shows how different cultural orientations impact upon concepts of health and illness and so affect how professionals and patients can relate to each other for better understanding and health care.

IV. *Cultural Influences on Education and Schooling* deals with schooling and the learning problems of children from cultural minorities within national schooling systems, but also sympathetically addresses the problems from the point of view of the difficult task of school administrators.

V. *Culture and the Law* takes up the different perceptions of culturally differing groups toward the legal system and the consequences in the legal processes.

Each volume in the Series has been written by an expert in the field who has had extensive experience in working with people of different cultures. Each has also carried out cross-cultural research in the field.

The books in the Series are designed for everyday use so have been deliberately kept to a modest size. They are intended to complement the accepted texts in the field and all assume the basic professional knowledge of practitioners in the field. Students in professional training programmes and participants in in-service development courses should also find these books helpful.

# FOREWORD

This book offers a path through a forest. The many and varied relationships between culture and health are what populates this metaphorical forest. At different times of day the light will play tricks on you with shadows pointing you to travel in one direction or another. These can be likened to the truly multidisciplinary perspectives that are relevant to an understanding of culture and health. While I have tried to be aware of these, the path travelled in this book doubtless reflects my own training in clinical psychology and my subsequent experiences of working in different cultures. As with any path, it cannot take in all that it passes by and so my description of culture and health is one which makes personal sense. The terrain covered in this book is not comprehensive, it is highly selective. I do not want you, the reader, to travel this path and believe that you have seen through the forest, but to retrace some of my steps and follow different shadows and chinks of light.

This book is written at a time of explosive activity in research and writing about both culture and health, and an increasing realization of the importance of their tantalizing interplays. I have omitted to tackle some topics which are undoubtedly important—emotion, interpersonal relationships, attitudes towards ageing and psychometric assessment, to mention but a few. Some of these issues are dealt with by other books in this series, while others would not squeeze into the confines of space allotted me. Some of the ideas included are, however, 'new' and doubtless somewhat raw. These include the

Problem Portrait Technique, the Faith Grid, the use of Critical
Incidents as a form of therapy and the suggestion of health
change progressing through Incremental Improvement. They
are served up to be chewed over and, if need be, spat out!
They are things which I picked up and put into my pocket as I
marked out a pathway.

It has been difficult to know how to refer to cultural group-
ings. One of these is the idea of 'Western' cultures. Of course,
there is no such thing as 'the West'. What is west of you all
depends on where you're standing. It can be the height of
ethnocentricity to talk of the Middle East or indeed the Far
East. If I say I live in the 'Far East', you may well ask where it
is that I am far from and east of! Yet such misnomers can be
widely understood summaries of an abstract concept. In this
book I have opted to use the term 'West' to refer to a range of
cultures which have some important characteristics in common. These countries include the United States of America,
much of Europe, Australia, New Zealand and to a lesser extent some countries which have been strongly influenced by
the values held by people from these 'Western' cultures. To
remind us that there is no such place as 'the West' I have used
the term with inverted commas.

During the writing of this book I have had the great good
fortune to travel five continents, work in three different uni-
versities and live in four 'homes'. The influences on me have
literally been too numerous to mention. The thoughts of many
people have beaten out my path and pulled back the under-
growth, so infusing me with the excitement and bewilderment which is born of true exploration. However, to move
forward you must have some way of knowing where you
have been. My editor, Daphne Keats, and publishers Comfort
Jegede and Michael Coombs at Wiley, have awoken me from
slumber when I have dozed off in some cosy corner of a
Malawian mountain or Irish hay field. Without the support
and thoughtful commentaries of my wife, Eilish McAuliffe,
and mother, Pat MacLachlan, the writing of this book would

have been a very solitary pursuit. I am also very grateful to Lisa Cullen for her skill and patience in producing the tables and figures in this book. Finally, a thank you to all those colleagues and friends from different cultures, who over the years have tolerated many strange questions. Some of your answers are in this book.

Mac MacLachlan

*Dublin, June 1997*

# 1

# CULTURE AND HEALTH

Multiculturalism is the only way in which the whole of humanity can be greater than the sum of its parts. If we are to avoid being churned in a monocultural 'melting pot' then this requires us all to acknowledge, tolerate and work with different interpretations of some of the things which we hold most precious. One of these things is health. The interplay between culture and health is truly complex and invites consideration of a kaleidoscope of causes, experiences, expressions and treatments for a plethora of human ailments. However, while cultural variations are intuitively intriguing and inviting to focus in on, especially in relation to health, they can also veil equally fundamental economic, political and social differences between peoples.

This book explores the complexity of human experiences of health and illness across cultures. The complexity includes the broader social context in which minority and majority groups operate. We must resist empirically stereotyping people as though they were 'cultural dopes' whose behaviour will conform to an abstracted 'cultural type'. Individuals must not be relegated to conduits of culture, but recognized as active sifters of the ideas presented to them through their family, community and social context, as well as their culture. Already we have taken as implicit some assumptions and definitions. Before proceeding further, the concepts of culture and health, which we are to work with, need to be unpacked. Following this we preview some of the main points of this book.

## CULTURE, RACE AND ETHNICITY

PADDY: *Good morning Mick.*
MICK: *Good morning Paddy.*
PADDY: *Ah, but its a great day for the race!*
MICK: *And what race would that be?*
PADDY: *Why the human race, of course!*

Ahdieh and Hahn (1996) reviewed the way in which the terms 'race', 'ethnicity' and 'national origin' were used over a ten-year period in articles published in the influential American Journal of Public Health. Their motivation for doing this was to determine the extent to which authors were complying with an objective set by the United States public health service, for researchers to explicitly refer to racial or ethnic differences in health status. They found that researchers only used such categories in their samples, either specifically (e.g. 'black', 'Chinese' or 'Hispanic') or more generically (e.g. 'race' or 'ethnicity'), in half of the studies. In less than 1 per cent of all the studies were 'race' and 'ethnicity' examined independently. Furthermore, less than 10 per cent of those studies which did use terms relating to race, ethnicity or national origin, explicitly defined what they meant by the term. Often the terms were used in combinations or interchangeably. It is also interesting to note that in those articles which did describe their samples using these terms, the majority of them did so only to control for their possible 'confounding' effects. Less than 10 per cent of all the articles treated these categories as potential risk factors in themselves. Ahdieh and Hahn concluded that there was little consensus in the scientific community regarding the meaning or use of terms such as race, ethnicity or national origin.

The idea of different human 'races' is something which many people are uncomfortable with. This is probably because it is seen as suggesting that differences between human beings can be reduced to tiny biological variations in nucleic acid. Furthermore, these genetic differences are understood to determine human behaviour in a relatively immutable fashion. It is assumed that if genetic differences exist, then they must influence behaviour. These possible differences are at their most controversial when they are used to explain variations in antisocial behaviour, intelligence or health, between members of different cultural groups, that is, when cultural differences are explained as resulting from different genetic constitutions. There seems to be an irresistible drive towards evaluating any possible differences in terms of them being 'good' or 'bad'.

The term ethnicity is often used to remove the pejorative use of 'race' and in recognition that different races may share a similar culture. Thus members of an ethnic group are seen as sharing a common origin and important aspects of their way of living. Essentially, 'ethnicity' refers to a psychological sense of belonging which will often be cemented by similar physical appearance or social similarities. This sense of belonging to a group can either stigmatize individual members or empower them through consciousness raising. Black consciousness in Britain can be seen as an attempt to empower members of a stigmatized minority group. While it is tempting to gloss over the sensitive issue of race its association with heredity makes it especially important to consider in relation to health.

## PSYCHOLOGY AND RACE

Rushton suggests that in zoological terms a race refers to a 'geographic variety or subdivision of a species characterised by a more or less distinct combination of traits . . . that are heritable' (1995, p. 40). He argues that differences in body shape, hair, facial features and genetics, distinguish between three major human races of Mongoloid, Caucasoid and Negroid. He further suggests that modern humans evolved in Africa some time after 200,000 years ago, with an African/

non-African split occurring approximately 110,000 years ago and Caucasoid split occurring approximately 41,000 years ago. Rushton suggests that the different evolutionary pressures produced by different geographical environments resulted in genetic differences across a number of traits. Through genetic drift, natural selection and mutation, particular characteristics were selected for in certain environments but not others (e.g. white skin, large nostrils), and because they gave individuals some advantage over those who did not have these characteristics, such characteristics later predominated in relatively geographically isolated gene pools. Thus populations in diverse geographic areas came to differ in their physical appearance.

Variation in gene frequencies may affect health in very specific ways. For instance, bone marrow transplants are used in the treatment of leukaemia and other haematological illnesses. National registers of potential bone marrow donors in Britain and North America consist primarily of, so-called, 'Caucasian' donors. Like blood, bone marrow comes in different types, human leucocyte antigen (or HLA) types, which appear to be genetically determined. Only roughly one third of potential recipients of a bone marrow transplant find a good match among their relatives, the rest being dependent on unrelated donors being identified through large-scale registries. Within the British and American registries the chances of finding a match for 'non-Caucasian' patients are considerably lower than they are for 'Caucasian' patients. Consequently, it has been argued that different ethnic groups should establish their own registries in order to improve the success rate for finding a matching donor (Asano, 1994; Liang et al., 1994).

There are, of course, numerous such links between genetic constitution and health. Another example is research suggesting that genetics may be relevant to the prevalence of Seasonal Affective Disorder (or SAD). SAD is usually taken to refer to the higher incidence of depression during winter months. It has been reported that descendants of Icelanders living in the Northern Territories of Canada have a lower incidence of SAD than that of either the indigenous population or of other settlers. In seeking to explain this finding Magnusson and Axelsson (1993) have suggested that in extreme northern latitudes, such as is occupied by Iceland, the propensity not to get depressed during the dark winter months may have been positively selected for through reproduction. Consequently the indigenous Icelandic population would have evolved with a lower incidence of SAD in northern latitudes. Further south, in Canada, descendants of these Icelanders would therefore be less susceptible to SAD than the indigenous population, or settlers whose ancestors originated from lower latitudes. This is a particularly interesting argument for us because it concerns genetic variation *within* a particular 'racial' group, that being 'Caucasians'.

Whether research bears out this 'latitude accommodation' hypothesis, or not, has yet to be seen. However, if correct, it would suggest that genetic variations are *not* synonymous with the traditional anthropological distinctions between Caucasoids, Negroids and Mongoloids. In other words, genetic variability is not a distinguishing feature of this classification. Furthermore, Haviland (1983) has also argued that genetic variation appears to be continuous rather than discontinuous. By this is meant that while people from different parts of the world may differ in physical appearance, no one group differs to the extent that different gene frequencies are found. Instead there appears to be a continuum of phenotypic expression, with different 'racial' groups to be found at different points along a continuum. Thus bodily shape does not change abruptly as we move across the globe, but gradually with neighbouring peoples resembling one another.

## FOLK TAXONOMIES

Physical differences can be observed in people from diverse geographic areas and these differences may have adaptive value. In the tropical regions of Africa and South America populations developed dark skins (densely pigmented with melanin which blocks sunlight), presumably as protection against the sun, while populations in the colder areas, such as Northern Europe, which are dark for long periods of time and where people cover their skin for warmth, developed lighter skins (less densely pigmented with melanin), presumably because they did not require the same degree of protection from sunlight. Fish (1995) argues that in some 'folk taxonomies' (local ways in which people classify things) light versus dark skin is considered a racial difference. However, Fish also emphasizes that other physical features that we associate with 'whiteness' or 'blackness' do not necessarily coincide with a black versus white distinction. He writes: 'There are people, for example, with tight curly blond hair, light skin, blue eyes, broad noses, and thick lips—whose existence is problematic for our racial assumptions' (pp. 44–45). Ironically the white versus black distinction is not seen as reliable enough to distinguish between people of different 'race' because each 'race' has a huge (and overlapping) spectrum of skin colours.

'Inter-racial' marriage further increases the overlap between the skin colour of 'blacks' and 'whites' and so to overcome this problem, in North America, 'race' has been administratively defined according to the 'one-drop rule'. If you are an offspring of one black and one white parent then you are black, in fact, if you have 'one drop' of 'black blood' in you, you are black, even if your skin is white! This identification of 'race' with blood is not a universal assumption. Different societies construct different definitions of 'race'. For instance, in Brazil racial categorization draws equally on skin colour and hair form, but may also be influenced by an individual's wealth and profession. This means that a person can have a different racial identity, not only from his siblings, but also from either of his or her parents too. 'Black' versus 'white' is simply one way of describing the variation observed between people. 'Tall' versus 'short' could be another, with accompanying 'secondary' physical and psychological features.

Indeed research has found that there are certain erroneous psychological traits associated with tallness (e.g. the impression of intelligence), just as there may be with skin colour. Thus people from different parts of the world differ in certain physical features and they also differ in how they explain this variation in human features. The construction of 'racial' differences in one culture can be quite different to its construction in another culture.

Whether there is one human race or several does not seem to be a crucial issue for health. What is important is whether there are some groups of people whose genetic make-up disadvantages them in terms of health. Such disadvantage will always express itself alongside skin colour, eye colour, hair type, height and so on. What we should be interested in is whether there are links between disadvantageous genes and the location of any individuals or groups on the many continua of human genetic variation. Such links, through providing physical markers for disadvantageous genes, can be meaningful and useful if they lead to health-enhancing interventions. Sometimes such links may coincide with skin colour and other times they may coincide with other characteristics. However, this book is based on the premise that the great majority of variation in human health is not related to genetic variation as such, but to the different ways in which people exist in the world, that is, to their culture.

## SOCIAL VARIATIONS

We have reviewed one aspect of our adaptation to different environments in the form of different physical characteristics which humanity exhibits; another aspect of this variation is the plethora of social characteristics to be found among us. Social variations exist because hunter gatherers in the Kalahari desert and car production workers in Tokyo need to organize themselves in different ways in order to get the best out of their respective ecological niches. Given that human beings inhabit many different environments and that human characteristics vary along a multitude of continua, it is not surprising that our social features, as well as our physical features, should differ around the world. The way in which we organize ourselves socially also has a form of heredity—a means through which such organization is passed on from one generation to another.

Harris (1980) suggests that what he terms 'cultural material-ism' is 'based on the simple premise that human social life is a response to the practical problems of earthly existence' (p. ix). Harris draws on Marx's idea that the means of production found in a society will determine its functioning, or culture. Thus different geographical locations will require different social orders (cultures) for optimal functioning. Social orders are passed on from one generation to another through a variety of mechanisms including traditions. Over the years people have organized themselves in certain ways in order to get the most out of their environment. Historically society has presented successive generations with similar problems. Social structures, from one generation to the next, have often adopted similar solutions to the 'timeless' problems of survival, for instance; food, shelter, reproduction. It is easy to forget this in our modern, ever-changing world, where many of us cannot keep up with the rush of innovative technologies which sweeps us along unknown paths. In the past, a social culture could provide solutions to the problems of living, over many generations. Such problems changed relatively little from one generation to another.

## CULTURE FOR COMMUNICATION

The term 'culture' has been so widely used that its precise meaning will vary from one situation to another. In 1952 Kluckhohn and Kroeber reviewed 150 different definitions of 'culture' and the passage of time has not witnessed much consensus. Some academics have tried to put the plethora of definitions into conceptual categories. Allen (1992), for instance, distinguishes between seven different ways in which the word 'culture' can be used. These uses are generic (referring to the whole range of learned as opposed to instinctive behaviour); expressive (essentially artistic expression); hierarchical (through which the superiority of one group over another is suggested in contrast to 'cultural relativism'); superorganic (analytically abstracting meaning concerning the context of everyday behaviour rather than the minutia of the behaviour); holistic (recognizing the interconnectedness of different aspects of life such as economics, religion and gender); pluralistic (highlighting the coexistence of multiple cultures in the same setting) and hegemonic (emphasizing the relationship between cultural groups and power distribution). Even this attempted simplification of 'culture' produces a rather complex matrix of overlapping concepts.

Here we emphasize a pragmatic role of culture, one which is especially pertinent to health. A culture presents us with a set of guidelines—a formula—for living in the world. Just as a biologist may need a particular 'culture' to allow the growth of a particular organism, social cultures nurture the growth of people with particular beliefs, values, habits and so on. But above all, culture provides a means of communication with those around us. Different styles of communication reflect the customary habits of people from different cultures. In each case, however, the culture is the medium through which communication takes place. A culture which prohibits communication has no way of passing-on its 'shared customs'.

At the most obvious level, it may be the custom for a language to be spoken in one place but not in another. A gesture may mean one thing in Ireland and quite another thing in Greece. An amusing example of this is the raised thumb used as a symbol of approval in Ireland, but as an insult in Greece, where it is taken to mean 'sit on this!'. Even in the same country gestures can be taken to have different meanings. In France, the ring sign created by bending and so touching the tips of the thumb and index finger, is interpreted to mean 'O.K.' in some regions and 'zero' in others (Collett, 1982). In a similar way a form of art may convey a particular message to one group of people and be apparently incomprehensible to others. Whether it is words, gestures, music, painting, work habits or whatever, a culture creates a certain way of communicating ideas between people. Culture then is the medium that people use for communication, it is the lubricant of social relationships.

Communication varies in many contexts. The form of communication may be quite different depending on whether you are at home or at work, with people of the same gender as yourself, whether they are elders or children, of the same class or caste, etc. We are each members of many cultures, or subcultures, as they are sometimes called. There exist subcultures of region, religion, gender, generation, work, income and class, to name but a few of the obvious.

It is the amalgam of these 'memberships' which constitutes the (often differing) experiences of oneself. This allows us to know ourselves in different ways. Different cultures require us to 'show' different aspects of ourselves. Different cultures, because they allow different forms of communication, allow us to relate to others in different ways and to be related to in different ways. Thus, experiencing a new culture can often allow one to experience a new aspect of oneself. Generally, we have most in common with people who share the same culture(s) and we find communication easiest (but not necessarily 'best') with them. That is, we share a customary way of relating to each other.

Not only is culture a 'voice' through which we can communicate, it is also the eyes and ears through which we receive communications. As such, customary forms of communication often 'frame' what we expect to see and hear. For instance, in one cultural context we expect to see a woman in a short white dress and people applauding (at the Wimbledon tennis championships), while in another cultural context we expect to see a woman in a long black dress and people crying and wailing (at a Greek funeral procession). Since smell and touch are also forms of sensing the world then they too are part of the machinery of culture.

Our senses are the instruments through which we receive and exhibit our own and other people's culture. What gets into us and what we give out (either knowingly or unknowingly) are the elements, or building blocks, of culture. When we 'just don't get it', no wonder things seem senseless, they are! Once the involvement of our biological sense organs is recognized as part of the process of culture, the psychological and physiological implications of culture become not only more apparent but also more credible.

## HEALTH: ILLNESS AND WELLNESS

Many people think of health as a lack of illness. This notion of health is encouraged by a purely disease (or medical) conception of health and illness. By this way of thinking, if you have an infection, a broken leg, an inheritable disease, or a latent virus, then you are in an undesirable state and therefore ill. However, a moment's reflection on this rationale easily illustrates its shortcomings (Antonovsky, 1987). We may understand by the term 'benign' that somebody has a tumour but it doesn't seem to be a problem at the moment—is this being healthy or ill? Somebody may be HIV positive but not show any symptoms of AIDS—is this being healthy or ill? A person who has experienced hallucinations and delusions, but who is presently free of them, may be diagnosed as 'schizophrenic in remission'—is this being healthy or ill? Someone who has suffered brain damage at birth may have reduced mental capabilities but above-average physical capabilities—is this being healthy or ill? The inadequacy of a healthy versus ill dichotomy is demonstrated dramatically by the brilliant Irish author Christie Nolan. He is constrained physically by a 'damaged' body but his intellectual insight and creative expression graphically demonstrate an unconstrained and 'undamaged' mind.

In 1948 when the World Health Organization (WHO) was founded it gave us the following definition of health: 'a complete state of physical, mental and social well-being and not merely the absence of disease or infirmity'. While this definition of health got away from the idea that health is an absence of illness, and that it is one (physical) dimensional, it has been criticized for the inclusion of the word 'complete'. As we have noted health is a multidimensional state. It can be broken down not just into physical, mental and social domains but into further subdivisions within each of these. We can at once be relatively healthy in some aspects of life and relatively unhealthy in other aspects of it. There is no clear line we cross to move from an unhealthy category into a healthy category. People, and their health, are more complicated than that.

In a subsequent declaration, Alma Ata, 1978, the WHO put greater emphasis on the social dimensions of health by focusing on primary health care. This declaration stated that resources were too concentrated in centralized, professionally dominated, high-tech institutions—especially hospitals. Instead it emphasized the importance of community participation in health care and the importance of communities having some ownership over their health services. In focusing on the primacy of the community this declaration allowed for the incorporation of community values. Different communities have different values. These differences often reflect different cultures or subcultures. Thus the movement towards community health also offered a mechanism for integrating cultural values into health care.

## COMMUNITY HEALTH AND ECOLOGY

In his book *The Psychological Sense of Community*, Sarson (1974) laments the downfall of the sense of community in contemporary North American society. A sense of community, or of experiencing a feeling of belongingness, has real implications for health. A considerable amount of psychological research conducted over the past thirty years has illustrated how 'people need people', not just for the sake of their company, but also for the sake of one's own health. A range of studies have illuminated how social support influences health, including physical health (Ornstein & Sobel, 1987; Uchino *et al.*, 1996), such that high levels of social support are associated with less stress, increased disease resistance, better adherence to treatment, easier labour and childbirth, less severe bereavement reactions and even reduced death rates.

As the importance of a sense of community, belongingness and social support have become increasingly recognized, health services have undergone a community reorientation. The ethos of community care has shifted our focus to the preventative, therapeutic and rehabilitative value of those people around us. The community is also the natural ally of the Primary Health Care philosophy. Around the world, in both the most industrialized and the least industrialized countries, for economic, clinical and theoretical reasons, health care has come home to the community.

Once again, if we turn to definitions we find that it is not easy to say exactly what a 'community' is. The ideal community, according to Heller and Monahan (1977) is 'one that maximizes citizen input by providing opportunities for individuals to participate and contribute to the welfare of that group' (p. 382). This definition of the ideal community emphasizes two important aspects. Firstly, 'citizen input' and participation are key elements in what has been described as 'community involvement in health' (or CIH, Oakley, 1989). Secondly, the recipients of good community health practices are the members of the community itself.

However, the community practitioner works in a context which incorporates much more than just community factors.

This broader context can be described as the 'ecological' perspective (O'Conners & Lubin, 1984), suggesting that a person's behaviour is strongly influenced by his or her surroundings. Thus while an individuals' personality, attitudes, intelligence and other 'internal' attributes contribute to their behaviour, their context, or surroundings, also have an important influence. The ecological approach therefore focuses our attention less on the individual's psychology and more on factors such as the community and the culture with which the person identifies.

This aspect of taking into account the person's environment is perhaps one of the reasons why the ecological (or eco-systemic) approach is becoming increasingly popular and effective in the field of public health. The ecological perspective, in allowing us to move away from focusing on the individual, allows us to consider whether 'the community' is a healthy or unhealthy organization in its own right. Winnett *et al.*, (1989) state that 'The ability to foster communities that promote health is dependent upon stimulating opportunities for group membership and influence, meeting group needs, and promoting the sharing of social support' (p. 130). Our conception of health now involves not just how the health of an individual can be influenced by the community, but also whether the community itself is healthy or not. These two notions are, of course, closely related, but not only in contemporary thinking, also among the ancients.

The origins of the word community are concerned with the idea of sharing a wall (Knight, 1994). A wall, of course, is a barrier; it can serve to keep others out, but also defines what is common ground to those within it. According to the ancients this sharing of space referred not just to physical space but also to the psychological space created by a sense of enclosure. It was not therefore only the physical space that was shared by those behind the walls, but also the psychological responsibility of living within that space and of being with others. Once again, in ancient times, such communities, often protected by a circular wall, would congregate for meals and ceremonial occasions in the 'forum' which was built at the centre of the community. Such a community therefore literally shared the same forum or 'focus' (a word derived from forum). Another aspect of the meaning of 'focus' is the fire at the centre (which people would crowd around). Such a fire could literally keep the community alive and meta-phorically keep alive the spirit of the community.

The ancients believed that places of great social value, such as a forum, were guarded by Gods. They would perform certain rituals in order to keep in good favour with the Gods. In effect they would cultivate the favour of the Gods. This was done by ensuring that only people who knew the correct etiquette were allowed to enter particular places like the forum. Thus certain rituals would be performed on entering a forum, and the performance of these rituals would signify the right of the individual to enter and take part in community activities. Such rituals and etiquette varied and distinguished one com-munity from another. The word 'culture' refers to the notion of cultivating—as in cultivating a crop—a relationship, not just with the Gods, but also with other members of the community.

Evidently the ideas inherent in the words 'culture' and 'com-munity' are intricately woven together in an ancient fabric of etymology. Of equal relatedness—and perhaps surprisingly to our 'modern' thinking—is the ancient understanding of health. Health was seen as an index of how useful or 'appro-priate' a person was to the community. It was believed that if an individual's behaviour was out of 'balance' with the re-quirements of the community then ill-health and suffering would result. Interestingly, according to this belief system, the individual who caused the imbalance was not necessarily the one who suffered. Instead another person, or group of people, could suffer because of the inappropriate behaviour of an individual. In ancient societies health was therefore a very public concern. How individuals relate to each other can therefore be seen to be a common element in ancient notions of culture, community and health. An understanding of how the self relates to others will be shown to be of crucial importance for contemporary mental and physical health.

## AN INTEGRATIVE MODEL

There have been numerous attempts to synthesize a comprehensive understanding of all things that affect health. Generally these models integrate physiological, psychological and sociological influences on health. However, to attempt this is no easy task and sometimes the complexity of 'bringing it all together' can confuse the reader. A model should, after all, be easier to understand than reality. Otherwise what is the advantage of having a model? Hancock and Perkins (1985) have described 'The Mandala of Health' as a way of understanding and remembering an array of factors which can influence health. The model sees human ecology as an interaction of culture and environment, incorporating a holistic view of health and recognizing the biological sediment of organs, cells, molecules and atoms which forms the substrata of us all. Figure 1.1 shows this model which, by its symmetrical design, implicitly reminds us of the importance of balance between different systems and subsystems. The community interfacing between the culture and family, allows for differences in lifestyle along with biological, spiritual and psychological experiences of life. These three 'divisions' are enclosed within a circle suggesting that they are often interdependent. Spiritual experiences may have biological and psychological aspects or consequences.

The Mandala provides an *aide memoire* but not an explanation. One of its merits is that it leaves you space to think. It cannot prescribe an action but it can guide towards a more comprehensive understanding, than might otherwise have been the case. The following case study provides a fairly tough test of the value of any model seeking to relate culture to health.

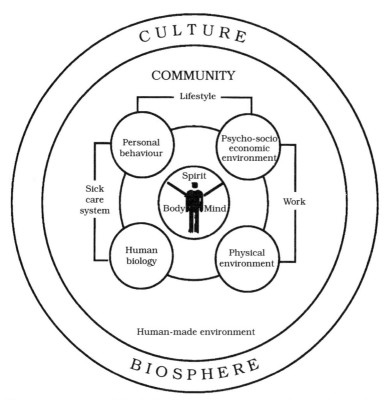

**Figure 1.1:** A model of the human ecosystem (reproduced from Hancock and Perkins (1985) with permission)

## Case Study: Torture or Tradition?

*In March 1994 Lydia Oluloro asked for 'cultural asylum' in the USA from her native Nigeria and Yoruba tradition of female circumcision. Lydia had been married to a fellow Nigerian, Emmanuel, who held a USA residency permit. Following their divorce, Emmanuel had failed to complete the necessary paperwork to allow Lydia and their two US-born children—Shade aged 6 and Lara aged 5—to remain in the USA. One of the grounds for divorce was given as Emmanuel's repeated beatings of the children. Lydia, who had been given custody of the children, saw herself as caught between leaving the children with an abusive father or bringing them to an 'abusive culture'.*

*Female circumcision is also described by some human rights activists as 'female genital mutilation'. Although the procedure itself, and the age at which it is done, vary across cultures, generally young girls have some part (sometimes all) of their external genitalia cut off. The clitoris and labia may be completely excised and the vulva stitched together. The girls are awake during the entire procedure, the purpose of which is to ensure virginity, reduce sexual pleasure and thereby make the girls better marriage prospects.*

*A.M. Rosenthal, a* New York Times *columnist, has called for United Nations intervention on the issue and for economic sanctions against those countries where the practice is common. She claims that many girls are left 'in lifelong pain and sexual deprivation' as well as 'more vulnerable to disease, infection and early death'. On the basis of Lydia Oluloro's argument, that her two daughters would be at risk of genital mutilation if they returned to Nigeria, the family was allowed to remain in the USA. In short, they received 'cultural asylum'.*

*Many African women living in the USA are opposed to sanctions. Dr Asha Mohamud, a Somali-born paediatrician working in Washington, says that 'The practice is not being done to intentionally harm anyone. Mothers do it in good faith for their children.' Alice Walker, the author of antigenital mutilation book* Warrior Marks, *has been criticized by Dr Nahid Tobia, a Sudanese-born obstetrician who works in New York city: 'It suggests, "I Alice Walker, save the beautiful children who are being tortured by their own people." It's like saying Harlem women give their children AIDS because they don't love them. In reality its more complex.' Indeed it is complex; some immigrants to the USA continue the practice of female circumcision, while others are disappointed that there is no formal provision made for it.[1]*

---

[1]This case study is based on reports from *Time Magazine*, January 10, and March 21, 1994.

Let us consider the utility of the Mandala for understanding culture and health in relation to each other. The Mandala model of the human ecosystem depicts the interaction between *culture*—as the most abstract unit of social analysis and *the biosphere* as the most abstract unit of physical analysis. As we have already seen culture and the biosphere are linked in that certain behaviours and social structures are appropriate to certain environments, but not others. The model thus emphasizes that lifestyles and community customs need to be understood in a broader context. Clearly American and Nigerian values may differ because they are an expression of cultures which have adapted to different environments. Instead of taking the context of an individual's behaviour into account, we often attribute the cause of it solely and directly to the individual in question. This is one aspect of the 'fundamental attribution error'. If we lack an understanding of the cultural context in which a behaviour occurs, then the behaviour may appear quite bizarre and unwarranted. The United States court judged that the Oluloro children should not have to experience the circumcision custom of the Yoruba. The court judged the practice to be unwarranted. It could be argued that the court's decision can only be understood in the cultural context of the United States of America.

Apart from drawing our attention to the context provided by culture and biosphere, the Mandala model also suggests the following sorts of questions (moving from the outside into the centre of the model) that might be asked:

- Does the practice have other functions within the communities where it happens? (Does it act as a form of initiation right into womanhood? What are the consequences of not undergoing the ritual?)
- Does it have an economic value? (Is a dowry system part of the culture?)
- How does it affect how females see themselves?
- How does it affect future intercourse and/or ability to have children?

- Does it have any spiritual connotation?
- Are there health risks?

The Mandala model is an aid to the community practitioner in 'thinking through cultures' (see Shweder, 1991) and in doing so being more able to evaluate and act in a culturally sensitive manner.

To argue that behaviour needs to be understood in its cultural context is not to argue for a liberal cultural relativism, where anything goes if it goes as part of 'the culture'. While evaluating cultures is a rather treacherous endeavour, I would venture that the value of cultural practices should be judged in terms of whether they serve their people well, or not. Beneficiaries may be at various levels, including the individual, family and community levels. If the practice fails to deliver some advantage at any of these levels, then it is likely to be of dubious value. If it is of value at some levels and not at others, then whether change should be negotiated or not should be judged from within the cultural system and not from outside of it. However, in the case study involving Shade and Lara Oluloro, a legitimate feminist argument could be made along the lines that 'leaving it up to the culture' would be to deprive these children of their basic human rights. This is an appealing argument but it must also be recognized as a culturally based one, even though members of that culture may believe their values to be 'universal' human rights. Let us not sidestep the issue here. There is nothing wrong with attempting to change certain aspects of a culture. That is how different cultures have evolved over many generations. Cultures will survive by adaptation but not by stagnation.

Airhihenbuwa (1995) has emphasized the importance of multiculturalism addressing itself to all cultures, and not simply the majority culture using the concept of multiculturalism to manage the health of other cultures. He has expressed justifiable concern that the agenda of health interventions is rooted in North American and European concerns to achieve what are seen within these cultures as positive outcomes, but which may not be seen as positive outcomes by other cultures. Whoever you are, and wherever you are reading this book, a cultural analysis of health is every bit as applicable to *your* health and *your* culture as it may seem to be to the culture and health of far off and exotic peoples. To understand ourselves, we must stand outside ourselves and realize that our way is but one of many.

We have now reviewed the conceptions of culture and health to be used here. Culture will be used broadly to refer to shared means of communication and social experience of living in the world. Health is seen as multidimensional with each dimension represented on a continuum, rather than in an all-or-none (healthy or ill) dichotomy. We shall place health within the community context, as this recognizes both ancient thought and contemporary practice. With these working definitions in mind, we briefly preview forthcoming chapters.

## Cultural differences

Acculturation describes the process whereby individuals encounter more than one culture and respond to the interplay between them in various ways. The way in which acculturation takes place, and the stress experienced, can seriously affect health. The reaction to acculturation is, however, not predictable and family members may have vastly different acculturative experiences.

One feature of encountering a different culture may be having to comprehend a different perspective on the factors responsible for health and illness. Within most 'Western' societies the biomedical model predominates. This model attributes health and illness to changes in our biochemical and physiological substrate, changes which often occur at such a microscopic level that belief in them is, for most people, an act of faith. On a worldwide scale faith in other causal mechanisms, such as the intervention of displeased spirits or the use of witchcraft, is probably more widespread. It would seem vital therefore to understand not only the nature of a person's presenting complaint but also their explanation of it, for the two are almost certainly interwoven to some extent. Health professionals, often through ignorance and sometimes because of arrogance or insecurity, may try to impose their own model on their patients. Clinicians are often less tolerant of ambiguity and less accepting of more than one explanation for illness, or suffering, than are their patients. Within a multicultural society, clinicians must recognize and show some tolerance towards a pluralistic approach to health.

In assessing any one individual there is always the difficulty of knowing to what extent they conform to cultural stereotypes. Stereotypes refer to conceptual and statistical averages, not to individuals. We must therefore find a way of mapping out how an individual's beliefs about their state of health relate to their own personal situation, the community they live in, their culture, etc. The Problem Portrait Technique is proposed as a mechanism for unravelling such interlocking influences. Through a collaborative interview methodology the clinician may assess the relative strengths of many factors which simultaneously influence a person's health-related behaviour. The Problem Portrait Technique is a way of integrating individual (foreground) and culture (background).

## Syndromes of culture

The idea of 'culture-bound syndromes' has been popular for many years. One interpretation of these exotic conditions has been that they embody social myths, perform certain social functions and/or reflect particular social pressures within the cultures where they are expressed. However, this sort of analysis may be made of any syndrome of illness. All illness, or disorder, occurs in a cultural context of some kind, and it is argued that, to some extent, cultural contexts influence the way in which suffering is caused, experienced, expressed and the consequences of such suffering. In describing some syndromes as 'culture-bound' it has been implied that some syndromes are not influenced by culture. Such an assumption is not warranted, and in most cases is probably ethnocentric in that it suggests that 'our' syndromes are not culture-bound but universal—that is, they really do exist!

If we accept the influence of social forces on our well-being then it follows that the problem a particular individual presents with may reflect factors beyond their self. An individual may, for instance, become anxious because of unease within the community they live in. In such a case a person's suffering can be said to point beyond that person, they may be a social scapegoat. If an individual's suffering sometimes reflects community or cultural concerns, how should this concern be demonstrated? What form should suffering take? A society which is anxious about the way in which child-like girls enter adult-like womanhood may express this anxiety through an individual adolescent female's concern with her body shape, size or weight. In an extreme case an adolescent female may starve herself of food, perhaps unconsciously seeking to retain the body of a child-like girl. Here we may also talk of the body being used as a symbol, symbolizing concerns within the culture. In this way cultural concerns may interfere with physical and mental functioning, either 'exploiting' existing ailments or shaping new ones into a form of cultural expression. The experiencing of a culture-bound syndrome by a person of another culture may reflect their anxieties over self-identity and cultural identity.

## Mental aspects of health

The cross-cultural study of mental health takes place in different forms. Comparative mental health compares the nature of mental health and disorder in one culture with that in another; minority culture mental health considers what the consequences of being a member of a minority cultural group are for mental functioning; and transition mental health is concerned with how experiences of, say, refugeehood or migration affect mental health. Each of these perspectives is quite distinctive but in reality they also overlap. Thus immigrants are often members of minority cultural groups and may be reported as having a higher incidence of certain disorders than the majority cultural group. A multitude of factors influence a consideration of mental health, and these factors should include social, economic and political forces which interact with cultural considerations.

It is tempting for clinicians to attempt to classify the unknown through diagnostic systems which are familiar to them. A Chinese person presenting with stomach aches, after experiencing bereavement due to the death of a family member, may be described as suffering from 'masked depression'. This insinuates that he is not suffering from the real thing but from something else which replaces it, for whatever reason. Contrariwise a Chinese clinician may say that a French man who is depressed after experiencing a similar bereavement is suffering from 'masked stomach aches'. Such an explanation would be unacceptable to most 'Westerners' because they assume the universal primacy of psychological processes. The only way out of such a riddle is to try to understand people's experience of suffering within the terms they experience it, that is, within their cultural 'terms of reference'. Failure to do so is to strip suffering of its meaning and symbolism and in so doing affront the integrity of the sufferer.

The communities which people live in should be seen as resources for community health. A sense of belonging and the opportunity to receive social support from people similar to oneself can have a positive effect on mental health. Also, residing in areas where the number of people who constitute a minority cultural group is large appears to be much better for mental health than living in an area where your cultural group is in a small minority. Such considerations may help to buffer the stressful experience of transition which many immigrants experience on arriving in a new country or culture.

## Physical aspects of health

Recent research in health psychology has demonstrated that psychosocial stressors can influence physical well-being in a variety of ways. The fact that many of the salient psychosocial stressors are likely to vary across cultural groups also implicates cultural variations in physical disease processes. As already noted with mental health, a strong sense of community, or cultural identity, may benefit physical health. Research on 'cultural inwardness' has found that mortality from serious diseases is lower where traditional cultural values are cherished. It also seems clear that some cultural groups live a healthier life than others. For instance, Seventh Day Adventists appear to live longer and have fewer physical problems than most people. We must therefore be prepared to learn from other cultures' healthier ways of living.

Reactions to illness will reflect the way in which cultures socially construct the meaning of illness behaviour. The Euro-American (racist) hunt for the origin of AIDS—placing it outside North America or Europe—may be seen as reflecting how Westerners wish to socially construct the meaning of a 'killer disease' as coming not from within but from outside of themselves. Whatever the origin of AIDS, clinicians have undoubtedly made some racist assumptions about it. Yet the complexity of this issue is evidenced by data suggesting that not only does the incidence of AIDS vary across cultural minority groups within the same locale, but so too does the mode of transmission and frequency of different preventive practices. Culture is crucial for our understanding of physical health.

## Treatments

One reason why cultures vary in how their individual members present illness is that different cultures require different paths to be followed in order to become 'legitimately' ill. To be a good patient in Brazil you must understand the Brazilian way of being ill. If the patient and their clinician each know the rules to be followed, then each can have faith in the other. The faith of a patient, or client, in a treatment is often referred to as the placebo effect. This effect applies not just to treatments but to clinicians as well. When a patient and a clinician come from different cultural groups this may influence the degree of faith a patient has in the treatment offered and in the clinician who is offering it. A *Faith Grid* can chart the interaction between clinician and patient.

Another aspect of the process of treatment concerns what sort of information is shared between clinician and client. Cultural differences in diagnostic disclosure (whether clinicians tell their clients the true diagnosis they have made) is an example of this. Patients and clinicians are cast in different roles by different cultures and this affects clinical decision making. Clinicians are a product of their culture and so too are their treatments. Sometimes inappropriate therapies can be oppressive. If a black person suffers from depression because of their experience of racism, then a treatment which focuses only on his depression (e.g. antidepressants or cognitive therapy) problematizes his legitimate distress. Such a treatment supports the view that the problem is with the individual rather than with the context in which that individual lives. The concept of transference can assist the clinician in understanding the personal history which individuals (both patients and clinicians) bring to clinical encounters of all kinds. Another technique which may be useful is the use of *Critical Incidents* as a therapeutic technique, whereby the clinician can help a client think through how the problems the client presents reflect their own values in the context of their culture. Rather than focusing on the culture and then 'zooming in' on the individual, the critical incident technique offers the possibility of focusing on the individual and then 'panning out' to take in their cultural and social context.

A recent development in thinking about culture and treatment is the recognition of the possible role of *culture as treatment*. For minority groups who have been marginalized by majority society, and who may in the process have lost any strong sense of identity and experienced low self-esteem, rekindling their culture, as a medium to their own rehabilitation, has been encouraged among the indigenous people of Canada and Australia. The current interest in the 'West' in different ways of living life (for instance, Buddhism) suggests that cultures, or subcultures, which are used as 'treatment' do not have to be one's own culture to be effective. The therapeutic effect of culture may simply be that it gives a sense of belonging—an anchor in the sea of life.

## Health services

Health services of the twenty-first century must adopt a multicultural perspective. These services need to reach beyond just concerns with the way in which different cultures experience and express illness, and how clinicians and their clients communicate, to include a community's infrastructure of care (of all types) in planning for health. Multicultural care requires 'Western'-trained clinicians to ascertain where they 'fit in' to the overall system, and not to centre the health care system on themselves. The community must be the home of health. Even in a monocultural society, clinicians of different professions will hold different (subcultural) beliefs about the mechanisms of, and remedies for, suffering. So too will the lay members of such a society. For their health beliefs are constituted from popular and folk beliefs, not just the beliefs of health professionals. As such the very notion of a monocultural society is a fallacy.

Greater tolerance of pluralistic approaches to suffering is now required. This tolerance must extend not only to allowing for other explanations of and interventions for suffering, but also to acknowledging that different systems of cause and effect may be synthesized in ways which do not always make obvious sense to you or me (from whatever our cultural perspective may be). This is not to say that 'anything goes', but it is to suggest that we should be open to empirically evaluating interventions which we may neither fully comprehend or recommend. In this sense, clinicians must be prepared to learn from their patients.

## Promoting health

Intervention can occur not only as treatment but also as prevention. We can also go beyond the idea of preventing things from going wrong to promoting things going right! For too long health services have reacted to illness and disorder rather than living up to what that phrase implies, servicing health. Unfortunately, even the best of health promotion initiatives are inevitably developed within particular models and cultural contexts. Thus cultural minorities may be disadvantaged because such initiatives are less accessible to them. Culturally sensitive health promotion will require working through different mediums and in different ways in different cultures. Flexibility and adaptability will be central requirements for health promoters working with diverse cultures.

Specific risk factors have been identified for particular disorders. In the case of depression, for instance, experiencing severe stressors, having low self-esteem and living in poverty have been identified (among others) as risk factors. The distribution of such stressors across different cultural groups may be uneven, particularly for minority immigrant groups. Once again we need to appreciate that cultural variation does not present itself in isolation from other factors which influence health. Cultural expectations may also constitute risk factors. It can be argued that the emphasis on individualism and achievement which is found in many Western cultures predisposes 'Westerners' to individual failure and self-depreciation, which may constitute a loss of faith in the self, a key feature in the 'Western' experience of depression.

Cultures offer different solutions to living and therefore different pathways to healthy living. They need to be understood at a systems level and not simply by extracting a few cultural practices to focus on. Health promotion efforts which do not acknowledge established cultural pathways risk derailing these important conduits of health. Clinicians, once again, need to see themselves as facilitators of health and not directors of it. Promoting the public health must be seen as a long-term strategic goal which will not be achieved in a biotechnological flash! Instead, such a goal is more likely to be achieved through slower *incremental improvements* in existing services, where the pace of change reflects what communities are able to absorb, while retaining their distinctive character and culture.

## CONCLUSION

The indisputable process of internationalization—the increasing contact between peoples of different countries—is often seen as making the world a smaller place, or reducing the differences between cultures. This is the 'melting-pot' perspective on our future. It asserts that the world's cultures will be thrown together with little to distinguish the behaviour of an Indian from a Spaniard, or the Irish from the Japanese. An alternative is the 'kaleidoscopic' perspective which is that we are not getting more similar, but instead more different. Internationalization is producing more subcultures within our traditionally recognized cultures. The Indian, Spanish, Irish and Japanese ways of life—the cultures—will still remain fundamentally different, as these peoples operate in ecologically different contexts. For some people this 'selection box' of humanity presents threats and problems, yet for others it allows a world of variety, stimulation and opportunities.

Many modern industrialized cities are thronged with different cultures and communities. A community is not a geographical location, it is a state of mind, shared by a group of people. You and I may be next-door neighbours, but inhabit quite different communities. Whether you live in Berlin or Brisbane, your mere physical location does not give you a right of entrance into a 'local' community. Your membership of a community will depend on your methods of communication, practise of rituals, adherence to certain 'rules' and so on. 'Mainstream' health services, and the clinicians who work in them, often fail to cultivate meaningful relationships with people who are not part of a mainstream culture. This book aims to outline ways in which good health can be understood and cultivated across cultures.

## GUIDELINES FOR PROFESSIONAL PRACTICE

1. The terms 'culture', 'race' and 'ethnicity' are often used interchangeably. However, they refer to quite different ideas. Race is, strictly speaking, a biological term and refers to heritable physical characteristics. Ethnicity is often used to refer to common physical features which are in turn associated with a psychological sense of similarity. Culture refers to shared customs of communication and common experiences of living in the world.

2. Variations in human physique are often taken as evidence for the existence of several distinct human races. However, it is also the case that human physique varies within the traditional anthropological categories of race. Furthermore, significant genetic differences may also occur *within* traditional race categories, and these differences do appear to be related to health. Consequently, while physical and genetic differences certainly do occur between peoples of different geographical

origin, the concept of race provides an inadequate framework for assessing these differences in relation to health.

3. Whatever concepts we use to describe human variation—'race', 'ethnicity', 'culture'—they are themselves a product of how this variation is understood to occur. Different groups of people have different explanations for this variation. As such, these 'local' ways of understanding human variation (folk taxonomies) are subjective interpretations. Different cultures understand human variation differently. What most of them do share, however, is the belief that their own interpretation is the correct one!

4. Human variation is also found in the ways in which groups of people organize themselves. Whatever form this organization takes, its functioning is facilitated by communication. In this book, culture is seen as the medium of communication shared by a group of people.

5. Our senses are the biological conduits of our cultural communications. There is no barrier between the psychosocial processes of relating to fellow human beings and the biological substrate of processing this information. Culture's influence on health is not restricted to mental functioning; it also affects physical functioning.

6. Health is multidimensional. It includes physical, psychological and social well-being. People can be healthy in some aspects of their life while being ill in others. On any one dimension, health and illness are not experienced in the absence of the other. Health is on a continuum, it is not a dichotomy. Thus patients are often healthy in many more ways than they are ill.

7. The community health philosophy invites consideration of how communities differ from one another. This is entirely consistent with examining cultural differences in health and recognizing that cultures operate through local communities. However, when considering cultural differences, the clinician should also consider the social, economic and political context in which culturally different communities operate. Sometimes these latter differences can affect health more profoundly than can cultural differences *per se*.

8. The belief that culture, community and health are related is not simply a reflection of modern practice, it was also a belief in ancient times. Our modern use of these terms often obscures their related etymologies. The way in which an individual relates to others is a common factor in culture, community and health.

9. The Mandala of Health is a schematic for thinking through and attempting to integrate the many factors which can influence health. It is presented as a clinically useful *aide memoir* rather than a comprehensive academic model.

# 2

# UNDERSTANDING CULTURAL DIFFERENCES

In this chapter we consider cultural differences in terms of human interactions and in terms of health. The social context of intergroup relationships can easily result in prejudice and racism. We consider how people from one culture may encounter those from another culture. Migration represents one of the most common vehicles of cross-cultural encounters. We review a model of acculturative experience which outlines the different ways in which immigrants can exist within a host society. The variety of cultures which are now found in many urban centres constitute a huge range of different beliefs about health and illness. We review a classic study of health beliefs across the world. Moving away from the diversity across cultures some psychologists have sought to empirically derive psychological dimensions which are common across many different cultures. Some of these dimensions appear to be relevant in areas as diverse as psychotherapy, teaching and physical illness. However, while large-scale empirical studies, and the models derived from them, appear to be useful at a broad level, they do not inform individual clinicians how they should respond to the person, from a different culture to their own, who presents an ailment for healing. The Problem Portrait Technique is described as a simple way of ascertaining the relationship between an individual and other social forces which may influence their health beliefs.

## MANAGING CULTURAL COMPLEXITY

To deal with the complexity of our world we naturally try to simplify things. One way of achieving this is to lump together what appears to be similar, ignoring (apparently small) differences. Sometimes we can get so used to seeing the similarities which we expect to see that we stop looking for— and fail to detect—important differences. In such cases the world can, in fact, become a more difficult place for us to manage, because we oversimplify it. The process of 'over-simplifying people' is referred to as stereotyping. Much of the psychological literature on stereotyping has concerned two related themes: 'in-groups' versus 'out-groups', and prejudice.

We tend to group people into different 'sorts'. People put into the same group as the self are members of our 'in-group', while those outside of this selection are 'out-group' members (Tajfel, 1978). Furthermore, we tend to differentiate between the members of our in-group, that is, we see them as 'people in their own right'. In contrast, we often fail to differentiate between members of an out-group. We see them as 'all the same'. In addition, we generally see in-group members as better people than out-group members. Research has indicated a number of ways in which individuals can benefit psychologically from identifying with the members of a distinctive group (Baumeister, 1991). A frequent finding is that group membership bolsters the individual's impression of himself or herself. However, and somewhat obviously, such membership is only beneficial if the in-group is seen to be a good group to be a member of. Groucho Marx's quip that 'I wouldn't be a member of any club that would have me!' reflects a crisis in self-esteem, not redeemable through group membership.

To feel good about our own group we elevate its status by focusing on the negative or undesirable qualities of other groups. This is referred to as 'out-group derogation' (see Branscombe & Wann, 1992, for an example). Thus for your own good, and that of the other members of your in-group, it is as well to concentrate on the positive aspects of your own group and the negative aspects of other groups. Out-group members are therefore discriminated against, even when there are few obvious differences between them and 'in-group' members. It is not necessarily that people consciously sit down and decide that the group with which they identify is superior to other groups, rather that in order to enhance and protect our own self-esteem we assume some 'natural superiority'. However, such a process of group identification is made easier if obvious differences do exist between the groups.

Cultural identity is often underpinned by physical appearance, dress norms, religious beliefs and customs which are quite distinctive. When out-group members look or act differently from ingroup members, then the oversimplifications inherent in stereotyping can be heightened. 'Racism' and prejudice may be products of the stereotyping process. From time to time we are probably all guilty of misjudging others, on the assumption that they are either similar to us, or different from us, on the basis of their cultural background. Thus 'racism'—or the negative stereotyping of different cultural groups—should not be seen simply as, for instance, the product of aggression bred of social delinquency. Instead, it should also be understood as a very common, if undesirable, 'by-product' of our attempts to manage a complex world.

Prejudice is as great a problem for the 'helping professions' as it is for anyone else. A true desire to help alleviate suffering affords no immunity from the psychological mechanisms which may oversimplify the sufferer. If you are working in a multicultural setting, then wouldn't you just love to 'discover' a set of rules (generalizations) for working with one cultural group as opposed to another? Such 'rules' would probably take the form of caricatures: 'Italians exaggerate pain—especially Italian football players!', 'Africans, being always happy, don't get depressed', 'Chinese somatize their problems'. Indeed evidence could probably be found to back up claims that 'the average' person from a particular cultural background tends to behave in a certain way in a particular situation.

The problem with this is that it's hard to know how 'average' is the person you are seeking to help. Thus the caricature 'solution' to working with people from different cultures is likely to build on our natural processes for simplifying and stereotyping. It makes individuals into what Garfinkel (1967) calls 'cultural dopes', who are expected to follow the rules of their culture. Unfortunately some of the cross-cultural psychological research falls into this category. What is needed instead is an approach to working with people from different cultures which will acknowledge the diversity, not only of peoples from different cultural groups or geographical regions, but also of the individuals within these groups.

## CULTURAL ENCOUNTERS

People from different cultures encounter one another in various ways. Historically, we have travelled the world for adventure, commerce, military and diplomatic reasons. In the twentieth century travel for leisure in the form of tourism has become more common. These days students also frequently have periods of studying abroad and professional workers take 'career breaks' or seek overseas work in order to experience something different. However, perhaps the greatest modes of intercultural contact are emigration and refugeehood. In some countries, such as Australia, Canada and the United States of America, immigrants far outnumber the indigenous people.

The encountering of another culture from either the 'local's' or the 'foreigner's' perspective presents various difficulties. Our discussion of the function of culture in Chapter 1 highlighted culture as a medium of communication. It was argued that such communication does not simply refer to language, or even non-verbal communication, important as these are in such encounters, but also to the way in which a person experiences the world in general, and the way in which other people experience and respond to that person. Bochner (1982) has outlined a taxonomy of the ways in which cross-cultural communication can occur. These cultural encounters can take place between members of the same society (for instance, black and white Australians) or between members of different societies (for instance, immigrants). Bochner also distinguishes between different aspects of the contact such as its time-span, purpose and frequency. Research has found that such factors can critically influence the behaviour of the parties involved (Smith & Bond, 1993).

We may have difficulty in communicating with people from another culture because they fail to meet our expectations:

> People are late for appointments, or early, or do not make appointments at all and simply arrive. People stand too close or too far away; talk too much, or too little, or too fast, or too slow, or about the wrong topics. They are too emotional, or too moderate, show too much or too little of a certain emotion, or show it at the wrong time, or fail to show it at the right time.
>
> (Smith & Bond, 1993, p. 177)

Smith and Bond suggest that such differences can lead to 'cross-cultural misattribution' where the explanations for an event given by a foreigner and a local may be quite different. Such difficulties in cultural encounters may have various effects on the individuals involved. A series of such encounters may give the foreigner some impression of how he or she is managing, or failing to manage, in a different culture.

## ACCULTURATION

Acculturation refers to the process of transition which is brought about by the meeting of peoples from two different cultures. Such transition may occur in either one, or both, of the cultures. Increasing internationalism and multiculturalism have produced a hive of activity in research and thinking on the effects of people from different cultures coming together. Berry and colleagues in Canada, have been researching a model of acculturation which considers the extent to which the newcomer modifies his or her cultural identity and characteristics when coming to a new country. The model is shown in Figure 2.1. It fits well the situation of an immigrant.

Although this acculturation model expresses the degree of cultural identity as a dichotomized choice, it should be thought of as along a continuum. The model (Berry & Kim, 1988) has been very influential and can provide some valuable insights into cross-cultural experiences. According to the model, a person decides whether or not to keep his or her original cultural identity and characteristics, and also whether or not to acquire the host culture's identity and characteristics (taking the case of an immigrant). **Integration** between the two cultures occurs when the decision is to identify with and exhibit the characteristics of both the original culture and the new host culture. Here the immigrant selects parts of both

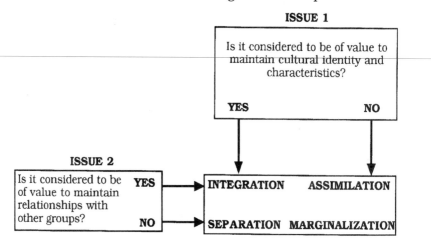

**Figure 2.1:** Different types of acculturation experience (reproduced from Berry and Kim, 1988, by permission of Sage Publications, Inc. Copyright © 1988 by Sage Publications, Inc.)

cultures and brings them together through their own behaviour and beliefs.

A second type of acculturation occurs when the immigrant
retains his or her original cultural identity and does not want
to adopt the host country's culture. It is important whether
this happens on a voluntary or involuntary basis. If voluntarily chosen then the individual is seeking **separation** from
the new culture. However, if this strategy is imposed on the
individual then the host culture is seeking to segregate the
immigrant from the main body of its society.

A third alternative is that the immigrant wishes to take on the
identity and characteristics of the new culture and disown his
or her original culture. This situation is described as **assimilation.** The coming together of many different cultures within
one society, where immigrants are willing to 'dilute' their
original cultural behaviours and characteristics, is sometimes
referred to as the 'melting pot' theory of acculturation.

The fourth option in the model is **marginalization.** In this
circumstance there is little interest in identifying with or displaying the characteristics of either the original culture or the
new culture. In essence, the person is living on the margins of
both the old and new culture. Such a person may not be
accepted or supported by either culture.

To illustrate the above four strategies Berry gives the example
of an Italian family which has migrated to Canada:

> The father may lean toward integration in terms of job pros-
> pects, wanting to get involved in the economics and politics
> of his new society, and learning English and French, in
> order to obtain the benefits that motivated his migration in
> the first place. At the same time he may be a leader in the
> Italian-Canadian Community Association, spending much
> of his leisure and recreational time in social interaction with
> other Italian-Canadians. Hence he has a preference for

integration when his leisure time activities are considered. In contrast, the mother may hold completely to Italian language use and social interactions, feeling that she is unable to get involved in the work or cultural activities of the host society. She employs the separation strategy having virtually all her personal, social and cultural life with the Italian world. In further contrast the teenage daughter is annoyed by hearing the Italian language in the home, by having only Italian food served by her mother, and by being required to spend most of her leisure time with her extended Italian family. Instead she much prefers the assimilation option: to speak English, participate in her school activities, and generally be with her Canadian age mates. Finally, the son does not want particularly to recognize or accept his Italian heritage ('What use is it here in my new country?') but is rejected by his school mates because he speaks with an Italian accent and often shows no interest in local concerns such as hockey. He feels trapped between his two possible identity groups, neither accepting or being accepted by them. As a result he retreats into the social and behavioural sink of marginalization, experiencing social and academic difficulties and eventually coming into conflict with his parents.

(Berry, 1990, pp. 245–246)

This quote also illustrates a very important point about acculturative strategy, which is that the acculturation experienced may not be the type preferred by the individual. The son wants to be accepted by his new culture, but isn't, instead he is rejected. This moves him from a preferred option of assimilation to one of marginalization. While the model seems quite appropriate to the situation of the immigrant, it can also act as a useful way of conceptualizing the experiences of refugees, sojourners, diplomats and others.

## HEALTH AND ACCULTURATION

Especially interesting from the point of view of health professionals is that Berry also suggests that the four different types of acculturation have implications for physical, psychological and social aspects of health, through the experience of *acculturative stress*. Cultural norms for authority, civility and welfare may breakdown. Individuals' sense of uncertainty and confusion may result in identity confusion and associated symptoms of distress. In fact Berry and Kim (1988), reviewing the literature on acculturative stress and mental health, have identified a hierarchy of acculturation strategies: marginalization is considered the most stressful, followed by separation, which is also associated with high levels of stress. Assimilation leads to intermediate levels of stress, with integration having the lowest levels of stress associated with it (Berry, 1994).

There is evidence that physical health differs across cultures in several respects. For instance, one study examined coronary heart disease (CHD) in middle-aged (white) males in Framingham, Massachusetts; Honolulu (Japanese-Americans) and Puerto Rico. Twice as many men died from CHD in Massachusetts as in Puerto Rico and four times as many as in Honolulu. In all three places cholesterol and blood pressure were related to the incidence of CHD. However, cigarette smoking and weight were not equal risk factors for all three groups (Gordon *et al.*, 1974). In reviewing subsequent research in this area, Ilola (1990) suggests that the changes in lifestyle and diet which immigrants experience may increase or decrease the chance of developing certain chronic diseases. In another study which attempted to link 'pace of life' with CHD across cultures, researchers were surprised to find that Japan, which had the fastest pace of life, also had the lowest death rate from CHD (Levine & Bartlett, 1984). Such a finding questions a common assumption that stress is related to CHD.

However, to complicate matters, Japan does have one of the world's highest mortality rates for stroke. This may be an example of how the experience of stress is expressed in different ways—not just mentally but physically too—in different cultures. Ilola also reviewed research which found that

Japanese men who migrate to the USA increase their risk of developing CHD, but reduce their likelihood of dying from a stroke. Such studies as these present us with valuable insights into health and illness. People who change cultures represent a potentially revealing natural experiment: they bring with them their genetic endowment evolved in one environment and then often adopt new lifestyles, diets, attitudes and so on, for coping in a different environment. In doing so they offer researchers a unique perspective in trying to understand the contribution of genetics and environment to health and illness.

I have only briefly described some stressful and damaging aspects of moving between cultures because this issues is dealt with in more detail in Chapters 4 and 5. However, it is important to acknowledge that migration, the adoption of new lifestyles and diets, as well as many other types of transition, need not necessarily be stressful experiences which interfere with health.

## CULTURAL OR CROSS-CULTURAL?

During the last decade there has been a lively debate concerning 'How universal is human behaviour?' The crux of this debate is whether some aspects of the human psyche are common to all peoples, irrespective of age, gender, class, culture, location and so on. In some respects the assertion that human behaviour is universal is commendable because it embraces the 'we are all the same and therefore equal' philosophy. Underpinning this argument is the idea that wherever people are, and in whatever cultures, there are certain basic problems of human living which they must confront. This is undoubtedly true when we consider such needs as food, water and shelter. However, it is also suggested that there may be 'universal' needs of a more psychological nature. One such suggestion is that how we relate to authority, to our own self and to conflict situations are universal dilemmas—that is, problems which must be confronted by every person (Inkeles & Levison, 1969).

The search for psychological universals is sometimes seen as a particularly scientific pursuit:

> Perhaps the most important objective of science is to discover universals, and in attempting to become a science, social psychology is in search of universal principles that can explain and predict the behaviour of individuals in all societies.
>
> (Moghaddam *et al.*, 1993, p. 43)

The notion that cultural differences in behaviour reflect different attempts to solve similar (universal) problems is certainly appealing. One of the corollaries of it is that different behaviours therefore have the same underlying cause. Some psychologists are so committed to this idea that their search for 'universals' precludes the possibility that they may be wrong! Smith and Bond (1993) suggest that cross-cultural researchers respond to inconsistent results in two ways: (1) sort out the studies which show the same results in different cultures and infer universal processes from them, and (2) consider the studies which do not show the same results and suggest ways in which the variations suggest universals which may not be immediately apparent. Thus either way—whether a finding replicates across cultures or not—universalism is the conclusion.

Another approach to studying people in different cultures has been to forget the idea of comparison *per se*. Here one tries to understand the meaning of a behaviour within its own cultural context, rather than by referring to a concept abstracted from other cultures. In this sense people are studied in their own culture, in their own right. To contrast this approach with the previous one, it could be thought of as 'we are all different and therefore equal'. Here, 'equal' means we should resist the temptation to understand the meaning of a behaviour occurring in another cultural context, by translating the behaviour into our own (more 'natural') terms.

By analogy, an apple and an orange may have similar needs (light and water). An apple and an orange may both represent attempted solutions, by different types of trees, to the problem of reproduction. But an apple is not an orange. Even so, we could describe an apple as the apple tree's equivalent of an orange! We could further build on their similarities to convince ourselves that they are nothing more than different responses to similar problems. Let us try to ground this in a clinical example. Brain-Fag (brain fatigue) Syndrome is found in several African cultures (Prince, 1989). It is most often found in very academically able students from very rural backgrounds, and is characterized by headaches, crawling sensations in the brain, blurred vision and various other symptoms. Its effect is to prevent students from studying. For the practitioner with some knowledge of culture's influence on health, it is 'easy' to see Brain-Fag as the somatization of a psychological conflict (say between modern and traditional beliefs), which would be more likely to express itself as 'depression' in the 'Western' world. Furthermore, amitriptyline hydrochloride appears to be effective in removing the symptoms of depression, for some people. It also appears to be successful in removing the symptoms of Brain-Fag, for some people. The practitioner may therefore conclude that Brain-Fag is really just depression. But is it? If Brain-Fag *is* depression, then why *isn't it* depression? Why isn't depression Brain-Fag and why are they different if they are really the same? In short, why is an apple not an orange? The fact that apples and oranges both respond to the same fertilizer doesn't detract from their 'appleness' or 'orangeness'.

I think I've taken the fruity analogy far enough. Trying to understand the processes involved in Brain-Fag by referring them to another problem which is possibly more familiar, say depression, is also trying to remove the cultural context of the problem. Illness and distress, be it anxiety or Alzheimer's, come about for a reason. In this sense the experience of illness and distress can be said to have a 'meaning' ascribed to it by society. If we believe that human problems have a 'meaning' then much of the meaning can be lost by attempting to translate the problem into a more familiar clinical/cultural language. Meaning can be present in the cause, experience, expression and treatment of a problem. As culture is a medium of communication, we cannot hope to understand problems presented in different cultures by stripping them of their meaning. We will return in greater detail to this issue when we consider the similar and more familiar comparison between depression and neurasthenia in Chapter 4.

## DIFFERENT UNDERSTANDINGS OF HEALTH AND ILLNESS

Landrine and Klonoff (1992) have recently argued for psychologists to give more recognition to anthropological studies in considering how people think about health:

> The major contribution of anthropology to knowledge of health-related schemas is that the health beliefs of professionals and laypersons alike are structured and informed by a cultural context from which they cannot be separated and without which they cannot be fully understood . . . White Americans tend to view illness as . . . an episodic, intrapersonal deviation caused by micro level, natural, etiological agents such as genes, viruses, bacteria, and stress. Thus, many White American laypersons and professionals may assume that illness can be described and treated without reference to family, community or the gods. (p. 267)

This could be considered to be the 'Westernized' view of illness and it is important to see this view as a cultural construction rather than the one and only truth.

In 1980, Murdock published his survey of 189 different cultures' beliefs about illness. He distinguished between 'natural' beliefs and 'supernatural' beliefs (of course such a terminology presupposes a fundamental difference between such beliefs, as well as reflecting a cultural understanding of what is 'natural'). He found that theories of 'natural' causation (including infection, stress, organic deterioration, accident and 'overt human aggression'), were far outnumbered by theories of supernatural causation. Supernatural causation was broken down into three categories. 'Mystical Causation' refers to illness caused by some act or experience of the individual as opposed to the involvement of some other person or supernatural being. This category includes fate ('the ascription of illness to astrological influences, individual predestination, or personified ill luck' (p. 17)), ominous sensations (including dreams, sights and sounds), contagion (coming into contact with a 'polluting person', such as a menstruating woman) and mystical retribution (violating a taboo; where the violation itself directly causes illness, in contrast to it being caused by an offended spirit or god).

The second category of 'Animistic Causation' refers to illness caused by a personalized supernatural being such as a soul, ghost, spirit or god. Included in this category are soul loss (the departure of the soul from the body) and spirit aggression ('the direct hostile, arbitrary, or punitive action of some malevolent or affronted supernatural being' (p. 20)).

The final category of 'Magical Causation' ascribes an individual's illness to another person, or persons, who use magic in a malicious way. This is usually motivated by envy or a feeling of effrontery. Sorcery and witchcraft come under this heading. Murdock's distinction between the two is that any person could attempt sorcery, while witchcraft is performed only by those who are witches, with 'a special power and propensity for evil' (p. 21).

In addition to developing this classification of supernatural theories of illness, Murdock rated the prominence of these causes across the cultures which he studied. The four most common across the 189 cultures were (in descending order) spirit aggression, sorcery, mystical retribution and witchcraft. Table 2.1 shows the percentage of cultures, from a particular geographical region, in which these four types of belief were rated as being ether the predominant or a significant cause of illness. As can be seen in Table 2.1, these theories of illness are not evenly distributed across the regions surveyed. Murdock provides a fascinating analysis of these results putting forward an appealing argument which accounts for the distribution of theories in terms of the psychosocial structure of different cultures. For the purpose of this book, however, his point is a simple one: 'supernatural' theories of illness are more common than 'natural' theories and they differ in their popularity across cultures.

## DIMENSIONS OF CULTURE

As long ago as 1935 Dollard was grappling with the problem of how clinicians ought to incorporate an awareness of culture into their practice. Dollard describes the individual seeking help as a palpable, concrete and real entity. The immediacy of the individual stands out against the abstractness and generalities of his or her culture. Thus Dollard notes that the individual always remains 'figure' while the culture is 'ground'. In other words, the individual is seen as the foreground and the cultural context as the background. The difficulty then is to appreciate the contribution of each, at the same time. I like to think of this problem as being similar to that of a reversing figure, where only the foreground or background, can be focused on at one time, but both exist together, and depend on each other in order to define their own existence. What we really need therefore is a way to see both foreground and background at once. The illusion is that only one— foreground or background—can be focused on at one time.

One interesting line of research in this regard has been to look for psychological dimensions which may be endorsed, to a

**Table 2.1:** Percentage of societies studied showing predominant or significant evidence of popular theories of illness in different geographical regions

| | Sub-Saharan Africa (%) | Circum Mediterranean (%) | East Asia (%) | Insular Pacific (%) | North America (%) | South America (%) |
|---|---|---|---|---|---|---|
| Spirit aggression | 70 | 96 | 100 | 92 | 63 | 91 |
| Sorcery | 57 | 23 | 26 | 52 | 83 | 68 |
| Mystical retribution | 48 | 8 | 21 | 36 | 46 | 9 |
| Witchcraft | 35 | 62 | 0 | 4 | 8 | 0 |

Based on Murdock (1980).

greater or lesser extent, across different cultures. We have already considered Murdock's classification of beliefs in the causes of illness. The way Murdock breaks down his categories can be simplified statistically. In an attempt to develop a questionnaire sensitive to different ways of explaining mental distress, Eisenbruch (1990), who has been critical of the dimensions suggested by Murdock, asked people to indicate the extent to which they agreed with the various categories given by Murdock. Their answers tended to cluster together, so that agreement with a certain cause was associated with endorsing some categories, but not others. Through the use of some complex statistics the way in which people answered could be simplified into two dimensions (see Eisenbruch, 1990).

Without going into the detail of these dimensions I want to make the point that complex ideas about the causes of illness can be simplified empirically, to yield a small number of underlying dimensions. The essence of this approach is that by knowing where somebody 'stands' on a particular dimension, it is possible to infer that person's answers to other questions. To return to the debate on 'universalism', a particular belief may not be universal but it may lie at some point along a dimension which has wide relevance. However, crucially for us, not only will cultures vary across some dimensions, but so too will individuals within a particular culture. An individual's rating on culturally salient dimensions will reflect the impact which his or her culture has had on him or her, with regard to that dimension. Thus, a German culture may not endorse the idea of mystical causation of illness, but the opinion of an individual German may not be that of the 'average' German. Thus individuals therefore have their own opinions regarding certain dimensions, within the context of their culture.

## HOFSTEDE'S DIMENSIONS

Let us consider the most influential of those studies which seek to empirically identify psychological dimensions relevant across many cultures. Hofstede (1980) reported the results of a survey conducted in 50 countries around the world. The survey had the advantage of all the respondents working for the same company—IBM—thereby reducing one possible source of variation in their responses (that accounted for by their work environment) not directly related to culture. Once again, Hofstede statistically analysed the data to try to identify any underlying themes, or patterns, present for the whole sample. He identified four dimensions and subsequently appreciated the presence of a fifth dimension (through examining the relationship between his own data and that of other researchers, particularly Bond's data). The five dimensions so identified were: power/distance (from small to large), collectivism–individualism, femininity–masculinity, uncertainty avoidance (from weak to strong) and time orientation (from short term to long term). In acknowledgement of the influence which Hofstede's dimensions have had we now consider them in some detail.

## The low power/distance–high power/distance dimension

The first dimension of power/distance is defined as

> the extent to which the less powerful members of institutions and organizations within a country expect and accept that power is distributed unequally. 'Institutions' are the basic elements of society like the family, school and the community; 'organizations' are the places where people work.
>
> (Hofstede, 1991, p. 28)

This dimension is concerned with how inequality is dealt with by society. Some social (or emotional) distance may separate people of different rank in the sense that a subordinate may not feel free to approach or interact with a boss. If this is the case—high power/distance—then a certain distance is expected between people of different rank. The dimension can be seen to be primarily concerned with dependence relationships. In low power/distance societies there will be interdependence between different ranks (for instance, through consultation); while in high power/distance societies subordinates are more dependent on their bosses, perhaps fearing the consequences of questioning or contradicting a decision made by their boss. Hofstede also provides an index by ranking countries for each of his dimensions. In the case of power/distance, Malaysia, Guatemala and Panama have the highest power/distance ranking, while Austria, Israel and Denmark have the lowest ranking (smallest power/distance).

## The individualism–collectivism dimension

Hofstede describes individualism as pertaining to 'societies in which the ties between individuals are loose: everybody is expected to look after himself or herself and his or her immediate family . . .', while collectivism describes '. . . societies in which people from birth onwards are integrated into strong, cohesive groups, which throughout people's lifetime continue to protect them in exchange for unquestioning loyalty' (1991, p. 51). Thus individualism–collectivism refers to the extent to which you act, think and exist as an individual (including your relationships as a parent, spouse or child) or as a member of a much larger social group (including extended family and community members). According to Hofstede, those who value 'personal time', 'freedom' and 'challenge' exemplify individualism. Alternatively those valuing 'training', 'physical conditions' and 'use of skills' reflect collectivism. Samples from the USA, Australia and the UK scored the strongest on individualism, while the samples from Panama, Ecuador and Guatemala most strongly endorsed collectivism.

## The low uncertainty avoidance–high uncertainty avoidance dimension

This dimension concerns 'the extent to which the members of a culture feel threatened by uncertain or unknown situations. This feeling is, among other things, expressed through nervous stress and in a need for predictability . . .' (1991, p. 113). People who are high on uncertainty avoidance are attracted to strict codes of behaviour and believe in absolute truths; they will dislike unstructured situations and ambiguous outcomes. High uncertainty avoidance is characterized by the notion: 'what is different, is dangerous'. Hofstede suggests that cultures high in uncertainty avoidance are characterized by active, aggressive, emotional, compulsive, security-seeking and intolerant individuals. By contrast Hofstede describes people from low uncertainty avoidance cultures as being contemplative, less aggressive, unemotional, relaxed, accepting of personal risk and relatively tolerant. Singapore, Jamaica and Denmark had the lowest uncertainty avoidance scores, while Greece, Portugal and Guatemala were the highest scoring countries.

## The masculinity–femininity dimension

This is perhaps the most troublesome dimension and for that reason difficult to understand. The basis for labelling the dimension 'Masculinity' was that men differed much more on the attributes of this dimension than did women. This was true across cultures. Masculine cultures are those which show the greatest distinction between men and women. In feminine cultures the roles of men and women appear to be less distinguished and more overlapping. This dimension might therefore be more accurately described as a dimension of androgyny, reflecting the extent to which there is a difference between the roles adopted by men and women. According to Hofstede, in masculine cultures men are expected to be assertive, ambitious, competitive, striving for material success and respecting the 'big', the 'strong' and the 'fast'. In masculine cultures women are expected to 'serve and to care for the non-material quality of life, for children and for the weak' (Hofstede, 1986, p. 308). At the other end of the dimension are feminine cultures in which men need not be ambitious or competitive, they may respect the 'small', the 'weak' and the 'slow'. In sum, masculine cultures are those in which there is a greater difference between men and women, while in feminine cultures there is less of a difference. Hofstede stresses that he does not advocate such differences but that his terms simply reflect differences in the responses of men and women in different cultures: 'it's not me, it's my data'! Now, you may wonder, which countries fall at the poles of this dimension? Japan, Austria and Venezuela were found to be the most masculine cultures, with Sweden, Norway and the Netherlands the most feminine cultures.

## The short-term orientation–long-term orientation dimension

This is the dimension derived from the Chinese Values Survey (see Bond, 1988, 1991). As the items in this survey were made up by Chinese as opposed to 'Western minds', this extra dimension, Hofstede argues, reflects a psychological dimension which is not easy for 'Western minds' to grasp. Initially Bond described this dimension as Confucian Dynamism because it related to the teachings of Confucius. Hofstede claims that 'In practical terms, it refers to a long-term versus short-term orientation in life' (1991, p. 164). He describes the short-term pole of the dimension thus: '. . . fostering of virtues related to the past and present, in particular respect for tradition, preservation of "face", and fulfilling social obligations' (1991, pp. 262–263). Preservation of 'face' (that is, 'face saving') refers to maintaining a person's position of respect. The long-term end of the dimension 'stands for the fostering of virtues orientated towards future rewards, in particular perseverance and thrift' (1991, p. 261). The 'top scoring' long-term orientation country is China, followed by Hong Kong, Taiwan and Japan. The shortest-term orientated scores were for Pakistan, Nigeria and the Philippines.

Before proceeding we should acknowledge that despite being an impressively large study, Hofstede's research has a number of important limitations. Most fundamentally there has been controversy concerning his naming of the factors arising out of his statistical analysis. It can be argued that the names given by Hofstede relate more to ideas familiar to the general public (such as the differences between men and women) or to researchers (such as individualism and collectivism) than they do to the statistical results of his data analysis. This is a crucial point because if the dimensions we use to understand cultural variation are a misinterpretation (or at least an idiosyncratic interpretation) of the available data, then they will surely mislead us. However, in Hofstede's defence it must be said that the interpretation of data (especially with regard to factor analysis) is to some extent subjective. Hofstede's work remains perhaps the most comprehensive study of its kind and a potentially enlightening piece of opportunistic research.

## APPLYING HOFSTEDE'S DIMENSIONS

The original four dimensions derived by Hofstede have been applied independently to the contexts of teaching and psychotherapy. It is useful to see how these apparently abstract dimensions can be applied to practical settings. In another publication Hofstede himself (1986) illustrated how the four dimensions were relevant to the educational context. Believing the teacher–pupil relationship to be an 'archetypal role pair' occurring in all cultures, he discussed how the four dimensions interact with this relationship. For example, in collectivist cultures pupils only speak in class when they are addressed directly by the teacher, while in individualist cultures they will speak up more readily in response to a general invitation from the teacher. In small power/distance cultures, when conflicts arise between teachers and pupils, parents are expected to side with the pupil. However, in large power/ distance cultures parents would be expected to side with the teacher. In weak uncertainty avoidance cultures it is allright for a teacher to say 'I don't know', while in strong uncertainty avoidance cultures teachers are expected to have all the answers. Finally, in feminine cultures pupils admire friendliness in a teacher while in masculine cultures they admire brilliance (see Hofstede, 1986, for a more detailed discussion of this). Hofstede thus suggests some ways in which his rather abstract dimensions have clear practical implications in everyday life.

Draguns (1990) has undertaken a similar venture with regard to the sort of psychotherapeutic relationship suggested by each of the dimensions. He suggests that individualist cultures favour insight-oriented therapy, seek distant 'professional' therapeutic relationships, and that themes of guilt, alienation and loneliness are emphasized in therapy. Collectivist cultures on the other hand would have closer, more personal and expressive therapeutic relationships, with a paternalistic or more directive nurturing stance being adopted by the therapist. Draguns suggests that the alleviation of suffering rather than self-understanding would be the target of therapy. Cultures high on uncertainty avoidance would seek the 'scientific' biological approach to mental distress, with psychotherapy being seen as messy, unpredictable and inefficient. By contrast low uncertainty avoidance cultures would encourage a plethora of psychotherapeutic approaches, with fads in therapeutic style coming and going. The high power/distance cultures would emphasize the expert role of the therapist, with therapy focusing on behaviour change, compliance with the therapist's instructions and on adjustment to social expectations. Low power/distance cultures would encourage self-growth, group work and patient support groups and movements. Finally, masculine cultures expect the therapist to advocate responsibility, conformity and adjustment on behalf of the patient, rather than the patient's own aspirations. Once again guilt would be a major theme in therapy. Feminine cultures would expect the therapist to side with the client against social demands, emphasizing expressiveness, creativity, and empathy. In feminine cultures Draguns suggests that the focus would be on anxiety rather than guilt.

Draguns analysis also illustrates how Hofstede's dimensions can be made concrete by focusing on their application to specific issues. Indeed by doing this Hofstede's dimensions have been made the backbone of 'Culture-Centred Counselling' which we will review in Chapter 6. There is also support for the idea that certain psychological dimensions may be relevant across cultures and that these are related to health. This research was also motivated by the reasonable belief that cultures differ in what they value, or believe to be important (Bond, 1988, 1991). Students from each of 23 countries (but note that countries are not synonymous with cultures) indicated the extent to which they felt different values (e.g. 'moderation', 'reciprocation') were important. First of all these data were collapsed together and analysed to find patterns in how the students responded. Once again two dimensions came out. Each of the countries was then assessed in terms of where the averages fell on these dimensions. Perhaps surprisingly, scores on these dimensions were significantly related to death rates from a number of illnesses, including ulcers, circulatory diseases and cancers. We consider these interesting findings in more detail in Chapter 5. However, at this point we return to the problem of finding an individual in the mass of statistical summations and averages.

## THE FALLACY OF AVERAGES

The sort of large-scale research, spanning thousands of people and many cultures, as described above has produced some fascinating results and spurred on intriguing speculation. These data may be very useful at the level of policy making but they have their limitations at the level of the individual presenting their problems to the community practitioner. These studies tell us about the norm, or the average, in a given culture. They are therefore a form of what we might call 'statistical stereotyping'; that is, they simplify (or reduce) the variation between people of the same culture. However, few people would be comfortable assuming the role of the statistically average Indian, Scot or Spaniard. While we recognize, and may take some comfort from, our similarity to other people in our own culture, we are also acutely aware of how we differ from those people with whom we have most in common. Our self-identity demands such awareness for without it we would be prisoners of our own culture.

Each person represents an amalgam of differing cultural experiences, to which he or she may give more or less credence than others do, and these experiences may relate to each individual's health and welfare to different extents. Each individual represents a unique interplay between culture and health. The challenge for the clinician might appear to be to decipher the extent to which somebody's distress (physical and/or psychological) is an expression of his or her cultural context. But this is not the problem at all! For in deciphering we are only translating a foreigner's experiences into our own, cultural, terms. We have already noted that culture is a medium of communication. Instead of stripping the client of his or her ability to communicate we must embellish the client's attempts to do so. The clinician must therefore find a way of understanding a patient's problems, in the terms that the patient experiences them. Fortunately, this is not as difficult as it may seem.

## PLURALISM IN HEALTH

It is very important not to make a dichotomy out of the 'natural' and the 'supernatural' cause of illness. These causes can and do coexist in the minds of client and practitioner alike. In

Malawi we have conducted a series of studies into the cause, risk reduction and treatment of a variety of conditions (malaria, schistosomiasis, epilepsy and psychiatric symptomatology) and have consistently found evidence for an ability to tolerate apparently 'contradictory', or at least competing, explanations of illness (MacLachlan & Carr, 1994a). This ability for 'cognitive tolerance' is not only relevant to health provision in the 'less developed' countries but in the 'more developed' and industrialized countries as well. This is because 'supernatural' beliefs also abound in 'developed' countries. A substantial body of research attests to the presence of such beliefs among Americans who originate from Africa, Haiti, Italy, Mexico, Puerto Rico, China, Japan and among the Native Americans themselves (Landrine & Klonoff, 1992). It is already the case that minority cultural groups within the USA have established traditional healing services within their communities. Reviewing the effects of immigration on the health services in south Florida, DeSantis and Halberstein (1992) noted that 'Virtually every type of traditional healer as well as complete pharmacopoeias of the health cultures in their country of origin are available to south Florida immigrant groups' (p. 226). The role of traditional health services and traditional healers is not restricted to traditional illnesses either, they may also have a role to play in combatting 'modern' afflictions such as AIDS (MacLachlan & Carr, 1994b).

Another obvious example of the coexistence of 'natural' and 'supernatural' theories of illness is when we attribute the cause or cure of illness not just to physical or mental factors but also to spiritual influences. In many 'Western' societies people sometimes explain illness and misfortune as 'God's will'. Consequently people will pray—to their God—for the recovery of a sick friend or relative. Although we may think of 'natural' and 'supernatural' causes of illness as being quite distinct, this need not be the case. We have recently reported a study of the explanations which psychiatric patients gave for their admission to Zomba Mental Hospital in Malawi (MacLachlan et al., 1995). Attributing admission to traditional factors was the most common explanation, followed by physical and psychological reasons. However, sometimes an explanation included more than one of these factors. For instance, one patient explained his admission thus: 'I was working very hard and getting quite tired . . . I had dizzy spells and my heart would jump and beat very fast . . . because of the success I had achieved, other people were jealous and put a spell on me' (p. 10). This quotation includes the psychological idea of stress, the physical notion of cardiac arrhythmias and the belief in magical causation through sorcery or witchcraft.

The reality of working across-cultures as community practitioners is that we are going to encounter understandings of illness and health which are quite different from our own. Sometimes our clients will adopt theories quite different from our own, and at other times they may adopt more than one type of theory to explain their suffering. To understand the suffering we need to appreciate the cultural context in which it is being communicated. We also need to hold back from automatically accepting assumptions which are a product of our own cultural communication and upbringing. We must address the problem of how we can 'think through', not only our client's culture, but our own as well. The need for this is illustrated in the following case study which is based on Sachs' (1983) book exploring how the Swedish health service responded to the health needs of Turkish immigrants.

---

### Case Study: Evil Eye or Bacteria?

*Mrs Mehmet, from Kulu in Turkey, has recently come to Sweden where her husband has secured a well-paid job. After several visits to her house by a Health Visitor Mrs Mehmet has been persuaded to take her children to a 'Well Child Clinic'. The doctor, dressed in jeans and a T-shirt, welcomes Mrs Mehmet by shaking her hand and asking 'How are you?'. Because the translator feels that it is unnecessary to translate this common greeting, the doctor gets no reply from Mrs Mehmet and proceeds to examine her 6-year-old son,*

*Yusuf. The young boy, cautious of the doctor, is encouraged by his mother to comply with the translated requests. While Yusuf is being examined Mrs Mehmet tends to her 9-month-old baby girl, Gulay, wrapped tightly in a large blanket, and resting on her lap.*

*The doctor asks Mrs Mehmet various questions about her son's health and she replies to them by addressing her answers to the translator. The doctor asks 'How is his health?' and Mrs Mehmet replies 'Good'. 'Does he eat well?' asks the doctor, and Mrs Mehmet replies 'Not so well; it would be good to get some medicine so that he can eat better'. 'Does he sleep well?'. 'Yes, fine' . . . The doctor shines a small torch into Yusuf's ears and nose. He then examines his throat using a spatula to hold down his tongue. He looks at his back and runs his hands down the boy's legs, grimacing to himself. Finally, he lowers Yusuf's underpants to inspect his genitals.*

*The doctor sits down behind his desk and starts to write out a referral slip. As he writes, he appears to speak to his pen, and says, 'Basically your son is in good health but I would like to refer him to a specialist in Stockholm for a second opinion about legs which appear a little bent to me.'*

*'O.K. lets have a look at your baby then', says the doctor as he get up from behind his desk and moves towards Mrs Mehmet and Gulay. However, Mrs Mehmet hesitates, appears anxious and tells the translator that she is just here for Yusuf. The translator tells Mrs Mehmet that since she has brought both children to the clinic then she must let the doctor examine both children. Uncomfortably, Mrs Mehmet allows the doctor to slowly unwrap her baby, revealing a tiny skeletal motionless body. The doctor cups Gulay's fragile head in his big hands, examines Gulay's neck and ears, and tests various reflexes, while rapidly firing off questions to the translator. The mother says that her Gulay has always been that way and that she nurses the baby herself. The doctor, beginning to appear frustrated, asks, 'Why haven't you taken her to a doctor before now?'*

*Mrs Mehmet starts to wrap the blankets around Gulay again, explaining to the translator that there is little point in taking her daughter to doctors because they would not understand what is wrong with her. Meanwhile the doctor, suspecting chronic diarrhoea and fluid loss as well as an upper respiratory infection, and fearing meningitis, announces that 'This baby needs immediate hospitalization!' He explains to Mrs Mehmet that she must take her baby to the hospital today and that he will telephone the hospital so that they know to expect her. He draws out a rough map of how she can get to the hospital from the clinic and recommends that she goes right away. Mrs Mehmet smiles gratefully and thanks the doctor as she gets up and leaves his office with Yusuf close by her side. They go straight home. They do not go to the hospital as instructed by the doctor.*

The encounter between Mrs Mehmet and a Swedish doctor reflects what we have described as 'cross cultural misattribution'. Swedish and Turkish cultures have different ways of explaining illness. This means that different actions will be motivated as a consequence of the experience of illness. The Swedish doctor wanted to admit Mrs Mehmet's baby daughter to hospital because he observed that she was underweight and had diarrhoea; he suspected that she had also developed a respiratory tract infection and meningitis. He attributed her symptoms to being caused by bacteria.

Mrs Mehmet had for some time been aware of the worrying condition of her baby, but she attributed the same symptoms to 'evil eye'. Furthermore, she believed that because the Swedish health system does not account for evil eye, it could not help to cure Gulay's illness. Mrs Mehmet is, however, familiar with the problem of evil eye and knows that it can only be cured by certain healers in Turkey. She has therefore been planning a trip back to Kulu for some time. Her belief is that her baby daughter is the victim of an evil force which is sometimes passed to children soon after birth. The evil eye— *nazar* in Turkey—is a notion common to many different cultures, generally referring to the evil glance which a jealous or envious person casts in the direction of the person they envy.

The glance has the effect of transmitting illness or bad luck to its recipient. It is believed that *nazar* can be transmitted by any person at any time.

There are various ways of protecting against *nazar*, of driving it out of the victim and of locating the person who transmitted the evil eye (Sachs, 1983). Of course, none of these readily relate to a Swedish conception of illness, and many Turkish people who live in Sweden continue to turn to their traditional ways of dealing with illness and adversity in times of need. These traditions are able to provide something which the modern Swedish system cannot: they provide an effective medium for communication and social regulation among the Turkish immigrants. If the Swedish doctor believes that he has a contribution to make to the health of Mrs Mehmet's baby daughter, then he is going to have to understand what it is that Mrs Mehmet values in her own understanding of her child's illness. We now consider a technique which I have developed which can assist in doing this.

## THE PROBLEM PORTRAIT TECHNIQUE

According to Chambers Twentieth Century Dictionary a portrait is 'the likeness of a real person', it is also 'a vivid description in words'. The Problem Portrait Technique seeks to convey a likeness of a person's presenting problems through both words and images. First of all we will consider the use of this technique with words. The Problem Portrait Technique (PPT) is simply one way of trying to understanding a person's inner experience.

The Problem Portrait begins with the person's description of their own distress, be it a broken leg, a broken marriage or a broken heart. Figure 2.2 shows the conceptual outline of a Problem Portrait (PP) for a Chinese immigrant to Britain who has been living in London for two years. Mr Lim presented to his General Practitioner with a continuous need to go to the

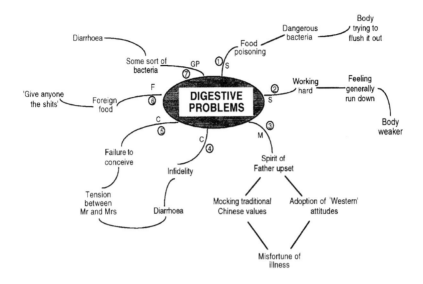

**Figure 2.2:** The Problem Portrait Technique illustrating different causes identified by Mr Lim for his 'digestive problems'. S, self; M, mother; C, China; F, friend; GP, most GPs

toilet, watery faeces and loss of bowel control. The GP classified Mr Lim's problem as Irritable Bowel Syndrome. However, in describing the problem Mr Lim used the term 'digestive problems' and it is therefore Mr Lim's own terminology which goes at the centre of the portrait. If a portrait is a 'vivid description in words' then they must be the words of the beholder!

## Causes

Perhaps the first obvious question is how and/or why has the problem occurred? What is the cause of the problem? The Problem Portrait is intended to give an impression of the eco-cultural context in which the person is living and in which the problem occurs. This means that we need to know the range of causes which possibly relate to the problem at hand. Firstly, as is good clinical practice, Mr Lim is asked for his own ideas about the cause of his problem. Mr Lim says that he believes that he has some form of slow-acting food poisoning and that there may be some dangerous bacteria inside his stomach which his body is continually trying to rid itself of, or 'flush it out'.

When asked what else might cause the diarrhoea Mr Lim suggests that he has been working very hard and feels generally run down. He speculates that 'somehow this can make my body weaker'.

When asked for other causes Mr Lim can't think of any. Now this may be true, but it might also reflect his judgement of the social situation: that this is not the appropriate place to mention other possible causes. Perhaps he feels the context—the often rather exacting relationship which exists between British doctors and their patients—does not give him permission to discuss other explanatory models of his problem. If asked 'How might other people in your family explain the cause of a problem such as this?', he may give exactly the same answer. However, the slight distancing—from his personal views—which is implied by the question might liberate him to talk about factors which he felt uncomfortable mentioning in his own right. For instance, Mr Lim may tell us that his mother believes that it is the spirit of his dead father, unhappy with Mr Lim's mocking of traditional Chinese values and his adoption of many 'Western' attitudes, that has brought about his misfortune.

In order to distance alternative causes further—away from the family—we could ask Mr Lim: 'How might other people, either in Britain, or in China explain the cause of something like digestive problems?' Mr Lim may feel that this gives him permission to talk about beliefs which he may possibly be uncomfortable with. This could be because he does not want to be seen to endorse them, but at the same time cannot altogether dismiss them. Other people may feel a lot freer to discuss cultural beliefs in which case such coaxing, or facilitation, would not be necessary. Mr Lim describes the belief, common among people from his region of China, that diarrhoea may result from infidelity, or the bad feeling which has arisen between himself and his wife due to their failure to conceive a child.

Mr Lim should also be asked about views he has heard from 'significant others', that is, from people who are in some way important to him. For instance, he may tell us that a work colleague told him that '. . . that foreign muck you eat would give anybody the shits!' Now Mr Lim may not agree with this view but nonetheless it could still influence him.

Clearly the list of causes can be long and their excavation requires careful and sensitive interviewing. For some people, explanations for their problems which arise though consideration of their eco-cultural framework will be easily discussed. In terms of a 'clinician as archaeologist' analogy, their 'social artefacts' are buried just below the surface. Yet for others their social constructions of reality may be much further below the surface, lodged in various strata of uncertainties or unwillingness to speak about things that you and I may not understand and may possibly even ridicule.

To conclude the investigation of possible causes and to appreciate something of Mr Lim's expectations of the consultation he is asked: 'What do you think that most GP's in London would say about the cause of your problem?' (note that Mr Lim is not being asked to predict what his own GP is going to say—again some 'distance' is retained by referring to 'most GPs'). Mr Lim responds by saying that most GPs would suggest some sort of bacteria as the cause. This gives us a range of possible alternative causes to work with. The Problem Portrait Technique presents the clinician with a complex outline of causal factors which a more conventional approach to assessment would have overlooked. However, those tempted towards a 'simpler' form of assessment—identifying the 'main' or 'real' cause—will simply be operating out of ignorance. If such complexity exists it is always better to know about it, even if it doesn't make your job any easier!

For each cause given, it is important that the clinician understands its rationale. It may be that asking for immediate explanation of a cause could make the person defensive, feeling the request for more information to be a demand for justification. Just think of it, most middle-class, white, British GPs are unlikely to ask for an explanation of the rationale behind a bacterial cause, but quite likely to ask for an explanation of how infertility can cause diarrhoea. It may therefore be better to come back to requests for the rationale of causes, unless, of course, they are spontaneously offered. Such requests for the rationale of certain beliefs can therefore be used as a way of legitimizing beliefs which the patient holds but is unsure of expressing. Alternative beliefs are often genuinely intriguing and simply expressing your interest in an open and non-judgemental fashion is all that is required of the clinician.

## Measurement

Although we now have a sort of 'word map', or picture, of the eco-cultural context in which Mr Lim is experiencing his problems, we have yet to identify what is 'figure' (foreground) and what is 'ground' (background) *from his own perspective*. The ease with which he discusses different causal beliefs may be no indication of this. We can however now ask Mr Lim to rate the causes he has mentioned. This could be done in many ways but the recommended way is illustrated in Figure 2.3. A brief description of each cause is written at the end of lines radiating from a circle. Each of these lines is the same length. Each line now becomes a scale of measurement (a visual analogue scale) wherein the strength of belief in each possible cause can be rated. The further one moves along the radiating arms, away from the centre, the stronger is one's belief in that particular causal factor. For instance, in Figure 2.3 'infidelity' has been more strongly rated as a cause of digestive problems than has 'working hard'. In each case it is of course Mr Lim who decides where the 'X' should be placed on the line in order to reflect his feeling about it. As in Figure 2.3 the scale may be made clearer by the use of statements 'anchoring' each end of one of the radiating lines.

Mr Lim could now rate each of the beliefs described previously. In doing this we can get an impression of how his own beliefs stand in relation to (his perception of) the beliefs of family members, other people in his community in Britain, people in China and significant others. We can also establish

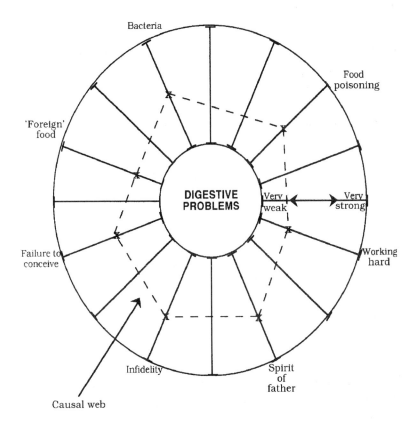

**Figure 2.3:** The Problem Portrait Technique for Mr Lim's 'digestive problems' with the strength of different causal factors rated along visual analogue scales

some measure of how tolerant of different beliefs Mr Lim is. If each of the lines radiating from the centre is made the same length (say 5 cm) then where the 'X' is placed on each line constitutes a relative ranking of the different causal factors. However, most importantly, this ranking is not presented in a linear context but in the context of multiple comparisons. There are significant advantages of these attributes of measurement when it comes to statistical analysis. But statistical analysis will not be necessary for the majority of clinicians who simply wish to use the Problem Portrait Technique to gain an impression of the range of causal factors and their relative importance.

Mr Lim can be asked to rate his own beliefs not only in the causes of his problem but also in each of their 'consequential treatments'. He could also be asked to rate what he judges to be the beliefs of his cultural community (or indeed any other party of interest) on these scales. The comparison of Mr Lim's own beliefs with his estimation of his cultural community's beliefs can help us to understand, not the extent to which, but how his own perception of his cultural background is influencing his own beliefs.

## Consequences

We might expect that beliefs in different causes are associated with certain beliefs regarding the appropriate treatment for the problem. For instance, the consequence of Mr Lim believing in a bacterial cause may be that he perceives the problem to be beyond his immediate control, and remediable only through the prescription of the correct medication by the GP. The consequence of the 'hard work and making the body weaker' cause is, on the other hand, that Mr Lim may be able to alleviate his problem through changing his own behaviour to reduce the stress he is experiencing, and therefore making his body 'stronger'. Mr Lim may also change his behaviour in order to appease the spirit of his father or ancestors who might have been offended by his behaviour. Another consequence of the 'father's spirit' belief may be that his problem is best treated by offering some form of symbolic sacrifice and/or prayers to his father's spirit. The 'social transgression' or 'infidelity' or 'infertility' causal beliefs may each imply different ways of putting the problem to rights, probably through traditional cultural practices, ceremonies or rituals.

The treatments described above may be referred to as 'consequential treatments' because they reflect treatments suggested as a consequence of believing in a particular cause. The treatment actually employed can be referred to as the 'actual treatment'. Thus the treatment which is explicitly chosen may subsume some, but not all, of the 'consequential treatments'. Indeed it is quite conceivable that the 'actual treatment' is incompatible with some of the 'consequential treatments'. However, it may also be the case that despite a strong belief in a particular cause of a problem, a person may choose a treatment which does not appear to be a 'consequential treatment' for their strongest causal belief. An example of this would be where a person believed that an illness was caused by their having a spell put on them, but that the best treatment to remove the illness is pharmacological, rather than one involving a spell of protection. Of course, it could equally work the other way round where, although somebody believes in a biological cause to their illness, they put greatest hope in prayers rather than in drugs.

We have now developed Mr Lim's Problem Portrait to centre on his own definition of his distress (or presenting complaint). Radiating from this are various explanations for these problems as expressed by Mr Lim through his own beliefs, those of his family, other members of his community and culture, close friends and Mr Lim's expectations of the sort of explanation which his GP is likely to opt for. Arising from these causal beliefs are various implications for how the problem should be treated, and we have given these the term 'consequential treatments'. Figure 2.4 subsumes Figure 2.3 and illustrates how Mr Lim's belief in the strength of 'consequential treatments' can be similarly illustrated. For the case of both causes and treatments a 'web', or map, can be constructed as a qualitative reflection of the relative strength of Mr Lim's beliefs. Such a map adds images to the words used in the Problem Portrait Technique and these images can help to illustrate the extent to which beliefs in causes and beliefs in treatments overlap.

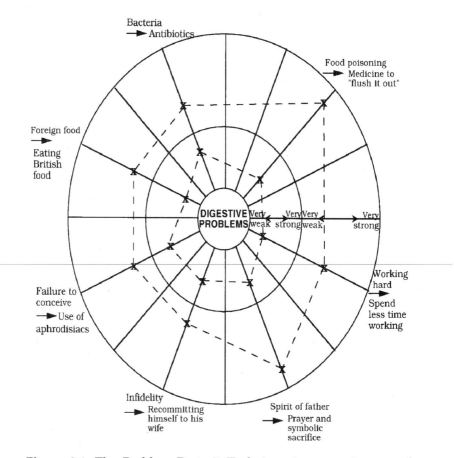

**Figure 2.4:** The Problem Portrait Technique incorporating causal factors and consequential treatments identified by Mr Lim for his 'digestive problems'

What I have described here is the 'Rolls Royce' version of the Problem Portrait Technique. Sometimes it will be possible to use the technique in its entirety, while at other times simplifications and perhaps dilutions of it will be necessary. Constraints of language, translation and time, to mention just a few, may prohibit the power of the technique. However, whether the version you use is the 'Rolls Royce' or the 'Mini', the orientation adopted through using the technique should enhance the quality of clinical assessment and therefore the efficacy of the treatment.

## CONCLUSION: WHAT CAN WE KNOW?

One line of argument is that if we study one illness or problem in many different cultures then it is as if we see the problem from many different angles. By taking away the cultural 'noise' we can reveal the true nature of the illness or problem outside its cultural context. This 'sterilizing' view sees the cross-cultural perspective affording us with a sort of psychological x-ray, penetrating more deeply to a common bedrock of human processes. Culture in this scenario is a *problem to be overcome*, a social construction to be deconstructed and outwitted, something which clouds the essential objective truth. An alternative view developed here is that different cultures create different causes, experiences, expressions and consequences of suffering, be it physical and/or mental. A complaint makes no sense in a cultural vacuum, because its meaning cannot be accurately communicated.

## GUIDELINES FOR PROFESSIONAL PRACTICE

1. Stereotyping, in-group identification and prejudice against out-group members may result from exposure to people of a different culture. Clinicians must acknowledge that their helping role does not make them immune from such reactions and that they, too, can behave in a

racist manner towards patients. Awareness of this, and acknowledgement of it when it happens, should be recognized as a key clinical skill.

2. Cross-cultural encounters are often uncomfortable and confusing for people even when disease and suffering are nothing to do with their reasons for meeting. Highly competent clinicians have human frailties, anxieties and confusions, just like anyone else. Clinicians may try to work through the anxiety aroused by some cross-cultural encounters by imposing their own structure. However, what is needed in these situations is *less* structure (compared to within-culture encounters) in order to 'free up' the client to describe their own problem from their own perspective.

3. Acculturative stress can result from the coming together of peoples from different cultural backgrounds. Clinicians should be aware of the effects which different forms of acculturation—integration, separation, assimilation or marginalization—may have on health. It is also important to remember that the acculturative experience of members of the same family may differ considerably.

4. Different cultural groups may respond differently to similar stressors and be at risk for different sorts of ailments. It is therefore important to be aware of health problems which may be particular to certain cultural groups and to be able to explain the reason for this both to the minority cultural group and to the majority cultural group who may control many of the health resources.

5. There are widely different understandings of disease and disorder and the meanings ascribed to them across cultures. The biomedical model, is, on a world-wide scale, a minority view. Clinicians should try to elicit the model which their client uses to understand their own problem.

6. Although large-scale cross-cultural studies have identified psychological dimensions which can be used to characterize different cultures, and these dimensions have been very influential in cross-cultural psychology, the dimensions do not necessarily apply to individuals. Furthermore, there is a danger of treating individuals as

'cultural dopes' by assuming that they comply to a statistically derived stereotype of their culture. The individual must always be seen as the 'foreground' and the context they live in, including their culture, as the 'background'.

7. Many people are able to cope with more than one explanation of their problems. Perhaps because they have invested so much of their own time in their professional training, many health professionals may be intolerant of explanations which do not coincide with the models they have been socialized (trained) into. Health professionals need to adopt a more pluralistic approach to health practices. They could, for instance, include traditional or alternative healers whom their client may also be attending in discussions about that individual's treatment. If a client is motivated to get an alternative and additional treatment from somebody else, then that practitioner may well have a useful alternative view of the person. This view should be sought out.

8. Being more tolerant of other explanations for disorder and disease may be uncomfortable for clinicians if they see this as challenging their own legitimacy. However, different practitioners may have equally legitimate, but incomplete, perspectives. Is there any one profession or system that can claim a monopoly on a holistic approach?

9. The Problem Portrait Technique is offered to help clinicians appreciate the many influences which may inform a client's understanding of their problem. It can be used to measure and weigh up these different influences and to relate them to the client's belief in different treatment options. Clinicians should use the technique in a flexible manner in order to facilitate the process of 'finding out' rather than to reach a predetermined treatment goal. The technique may be especially useful for identifying alternative treatments that could be used simultaneously.

10. Clinicians working across cultures should not try to strip away the confounding effects of culture in order to understand their clients better, but should try to explore how their clients use their culture as a medium of communication through which to express their suffering.

# 3

# CULTURE-BOUND SYNDROMES

It has already been emphasized that many major cities are now home to a great range of cultural groups and, as such, the ailments presented to clinicians are much more diverse than ever before, at least in urban areas. A French community nurse at the turn of this century may encounter forms of suffering only known to specialists in tropical medicine at the turn of the last century. It is easy to alienate oneself from this baffling array of foreign disorders, seeing them, for instance, as the 'cultural baggage' of immigrants. One way in which this alienation can unintentionally occur is through our assumptions about what constitutes a 'culture-bound syndrome' and what doesn't. In this chapter we consider to what extent any, or all, forms of suffering can be considered 'culture bound'. We will pay specific attention to understanding the social function of human suffering. We also look at the extent to which culture 'exploits' universal phenomena on the one hand and, on the other, the extent to which it sculptures forms of suffering out of the social and environmental fabric which different cultures provide. By turning this form of analysis on European peoples too we consider to what extent 'Western' disorders are bounded by 'Western' cultures. The chapter ends with some guidelines on how to think through the role of culture in the causes, experience, expression and consequence of human suffering.

## SANTA CLAUS: MORE THAN JUST GOOD FUN

When we consider the diversity of beliefs across different cultures it is important to look at the consequences of the beliefs within the culture in which they are held. If we think of cultural beliefs as part of a broader process of communication within the culture then we can begin to understand what functions are served by a particular belief system. Consider, for instance, the popular 'Western' belief in Santa Claus. This is an interesting belief for many reasons. Children tend to be the strongest believers, and are encouraged in their belief by adults. Although adults tend not to believe in Santa Claus, they often behave as though they do and will even act out his role in order to perpetuate the myth. Children who have themselves discovered that Santa is not 'real' will often go along with the notion in order to retain the magic of the myth for younger children.

What is the function of the Santa Claus myth? Let's consider just one interpretation. As already mentioned, children may be educated, or socialized, into believing in Santa Claus. We understand him to be a cheerful old man with a large white beard who will give us presents at Christmas time if we are good. Santa Claus, apart from being good fun or perhaps because he is good fun, can also be seen as having a social regulatory function on children growing up. Through Santa they may learn to respect older people, see them as kind and be encouraged to behave according to certain rules or norms, in order to be rewarded. These ideas, among others, are communicated to us through the vehicle of Santa Claus. If we get the message, then we get the present!

It is not, of course, that the idea of Santa is part of some devious plot to control little children (although many such plots doubtless exist!), but instead that the notion of Santa Claus has been used (selected) across many generations (of parents) because it has some social benefits, as well as being good fun. The social function of Santa is also apparent in our choice of him being old, bearded and plump. We have not chosen to endorse alternative images of Santa. He is not presented as a reformed alcoholic or a mini-skirted blonde in stiletto heels. Either of these figures could just as easily be the bearer of gifts to our children in reward for their good behaviour. However, they are not. Santa Claus cultures don't want to communicate those messages. It can therefore be seen that the myth of Santa is not an arbitrary idea; it has not just been chosen at random for its 'feel good' factor.

At least some of the beliefs which a society encourages its members to adopt can be seen to have a regulatory function for the society. I have focused on the idea of Santa Claus as just one example of a general principle and given only one interpretation of the Santa Claus myth. Sorry if I'm the first to break the news to you! Other ideas—God, nuclear explosions and prisoners on 'death row'—can also be analysed in terms of their having a social function and a social construction. However, it often seems easier to analyse the social function of a myth than the social function of a reality. Perhaps this is because if we know something to be a myth we can then ask 'What is the function of this idea?', based on the assumption that if the idea didn't have a function then it wouldn't continue to exist.

Something which is a reality can also serve a social function. Real events may take on 'mythical' significance. Cancer, AIDS and heart disease are all illnesses around which myths have built up. Indeed the greater the basis of an idea in reality—for instance, that AIDS is incurable—then the stronger a vehicle it may be to transmit ideas which are myths: 'AIDS is a punishment from God for promiscuity.' While one possible regulatory function of this belief—to reduce promiscuity—may be rather obvious, many health beliefs have more subtle functions.

## CULTURE BOUND OR CONCEPT BOUND?

Before we consider two of the classic 'culture-bound syndromes' let us consider in more detail the very term 'culture bound'. Specifically let us from the outset acknowledge the ethnocentricity of the very term 'culture bound'. Essentially this term is used to describe disorders or illnesses with which the people making the classification are not familiar. For instance, Margaret Clark (1985) has described the problem of 'latido' in a community of Mexican-Americans. Latido is characterized by significant weakness, abdominal pulsations and emaciation brought on by the victim being unable to eat. Because this array of symptoms is not familiar to us, yet occurs in sufficient cluster to be called a syndrome, it is described as a condition found within the bounds of another culture.

If we stop to think about it for a moment we realize that some of the conditions which we may accept as universal (or 'non-culture bound'), say anorexia nervosa or obesity, may simply be bound by our own culture. Once again, looking across cultures may allow us to view our own culture in clearer perspective. It may also lead us to review our concept of some syndromes being 'culture bound' and others being 'un-culture bound', or universal.

There is without doubt something intuitively appealing about the 'dramatic exotica' (Simons, 1985, p. 43) which culture-bound syndromes represent. It is important to view these problems not in a voyeuristic fashion but to see beyond the 'colourful display' and understand the social meaning and function of the disorder. After all, a Martian who happened to be looking in on your house on Christmas Eve could come away with a rather bizarre impression of human behaviour, unless it understood the context in which the bearded man in red costume was hanging (handling!) a stocking above a little girl's bed!

The two syndromes which we will now consider, koro and latah, have been chosen to illustrate particular points. In describing koro I will pay particular attention to demonstrating how apparently bizarre behaviour can be understood to have both an *order* and a *function*, when presented in the context of salient cultural beliefs. The second syndrome, latah, will help to illustrate the intricacies of debates concerning the ways in which 'culture-bound syndromes' are related to culture. To understand and assist people who present problems which are foreign to us, it is important to be aware of these two issues.

## KORO

Koro is a condition where people believe that their sexual organs are shrinking. It is believed to be a fatal condition and occurs mostly in southern China and Southeast Asia (Cheng, 1994). Although it usually occurs in isolated cases, epidemics of koro may also occur. It is, of course, natural to try to understand new problems by classifying them into more familiar ways of seeing the world. Thus koro, in terms of 'Western' diagnostic criteria, has been subsumed as a variant of dissociative disorder, somatoform disorder, panic disorder and even psychosis.

Koro is most commonly associated with males through their fear of penis shrinkage. In fact, although it is much less common in females, it is also found in women as a fear of retracting nipples, breasts or labia. For both sexes the fear of shrinkage is associated with the fear of imminent death, the shrinkage being only a precursor to this. Cheng (1994, pp. 7–8) gives a vivid description of the onset of koro:

> Usually, the malady begins with a feeling on the part of the victim that his or her sex organ is shrinking. Believing that the condition is critical, the victim becomes extremely anxious, doing whatever he or she can to stop the sex organ from further retracting and crying vigorously for help. A man may be seen holding his penis, 'anchoring' it with some clamping device, or tying the penis with a piece of string. Similarly a woman may be seen grabbing her own breasts, pulling her nipples, or even having iron pins

inserted through the nipples, all to prevent the retraction of the respective organs.

The process of rescuing the organs may look highly absurd to an outsider, even to a Chinese. Imagine someone shouting for help and at the same time pulling his or her genital, thus exposing it, in public. The victim's relatives and neighbours will rush to 'help out' because they too believe that the condition can be fatal. . . . In fact, many so-called 'patients' were diagnosed with Koro not because they themselves had initiated the complaint, but because other people around them had misinterpreted signs of discomfort to mean Koro and performed the rescue. . . . For example, . . . a bride was thought to have Koro on the wedding day because she appeared pale and weak. The rescue effort continued for a while until she yelled out that she was not experiencing breast shrinkage!

Such behaviour may indeed seem absurd to us. Does it still seem absurd if we consider its sociocultural context? Attempts to rescue a person suspected of having koro are so strenuous because a person with koro is seen as a dying person. Everybody of the same sex as the victim (the social norm is that only members of the same sex can attempt to rescue a victim) in the vicinity will rush to help the person suspected of having koro. Their efforts will continue until everyone gets exhausted and anxiety about the victim's imminent death subsides.

To diagnose this condition purely in terms of its symptoms— suspected organ shrinkage, pale complexion, shivering, hyperventilation, palpitations, sweating, fainting, etc.—would be quite insufficient. We can only meaningfully classify it if we understand it. Cheng's (1994) study of koro found that it is most common among adolescent males who are single, poorly educated, lacking (alternative) sexual knowledge and who had a strong belief in the notion of koro. From the perspective of this book, koro is an especially interesting phenomenon because, as Cheng argues, it cannot be understood from the perspective of the individual's (psycho)pathology but rather as an expression of a *community's* anxiety.

Cheng provides us with information on the cultural context in which koro occurs. The notion of sexual restraint is prominent in Chinese cultures. The amount of semen which a man can produce is understood to be limited. It is considered to be a man's 'vital energy' and must therefore be used economically; sexual intercourse resulting in ejaculation should only occur when the woman is ovulating. The notion that death can result from a depletion of semen may be an important background factor in koro, because it relates sexuality to death.

A second thread to this complex fabric of understanding the sociocultural context of koro comes from the Chinese folklore of the 'fox spirit' which can seduce people, sap their 'vital energy' and thereby make them weak. The 'fox spirit' is able to shrink tissue and this provides a direct link, in folklore, to koro. It does not, however, explain the social function of koro.

A community may come to expect or experience misfortune in, for instance, its (agricultural) production or the health of its members. The 'fox spirit', it is believed, roams the world in search of victims. When things are not going well this may be taken as an indication that the 'fox spirit' has visited a community. A fortune teller's prediction of its visitation will create considerable uncertainty and anxiety. The community becomes hypervigilant to detect the first arrival of the 'fox spirit'. Cheng suggests that the failure to identify any objective signs of a ghost heightens tension to such a degree that victimization becomes an inevitable outlet for the community's anxiety.

An individual's behaviour may lead others to 'realize' that the person is suffering from a koro attack. On the other hand, an individual himself may suspect a koro attack is beginning (cold sensations or insect bites in the genital area which can temporarily reduce the size of the genitalia, along with weakness or sickness, may be interpreted as the onset of an attack). Through the identification of a victim the anxiety of the whole community may be relieved. As people rush to help rescue the victim, the failure of the victim's genitalia to truly retract is taken as evidence that the 'fox spirit' has been exorcized and moved on. The community is thus saved, tension reduced and effort may be turned to overcoming other problems, be they health or crop production. Once the spirit has visited a community and moved on it should not return for some time.

The above is only one interpretation of the koro syndrome and a simplified one at that. Nonetheless is does stand to illustrate how koro can be understood in terms of the sociocultural context in which it occurs. In this context it is an *ordered* and *functional* phenomenon: it occurs in a particular way which makes sense (order) and it has a purpose (function). Koro is a vehicle through which the community can communicate its anxiety and engineer its own cure. Naturally, individual members of the community may not interpret koro in this manner. To them it will be a frightening reality to be avoided at all costs. A visitation of death to be escaped.

When an individual holds such an understanding of their own experience and presents it to a clinician in a foreign land, then the challenge for the clinician is to hold back from assuming a cure and learn about its cause and function. Only through such an approach can the concerns of the patient be truly relieved. It has been assumed by many 'Western' clinicians that the longer minority cultural groups stay in 'Western' countries the less they will present problems arising from their own cultural heritage. It is now becoming clear that this is not going to be the case. People define themselves in relation to their family, friends, communities and so on. These are the vehicles of culture. It is now recognized that tolerance towards ethnic differences is to be valued and encouraged. Social legislation across the European Union, America, Australia and other traditionally 'Western' countries explicitly states this. Many clinicians may need to adapt their perspective on health and culture if they are to be of service to the array of people within their own communities. Koro demonstrates how understanding the cultural context demystifies certain behaviours. Latah also illustrates this point.

## LATAH

Latah is another syndrome found in Malaysia and Indonesia. It is characterized by an exaggerated startled response to a surprising event. This response may take the form of throwing or dropping an object which was being held and the utterance of rude words, such as 'puki!' ('cunt!'), 'butol!' ('prick!') or 'buntut!' ('arse!') (Simons, 1985, p. 43). The startled person may also, apparently automatically, carry out instructions given by somebody close by, or mimic the words or movements of someone nearby at the time of the startle. The spectators of such behaviour are usually amused by it and this may lead a known latah to be intentionally startled (perhaps several times a day) in order to amuse others.

Latah may develop into a life-long condition regardless of whether its onset is abrupt or gradual. It is found in both men and women, being most common in middle-aged women of low social status. While common in some families, it also occurs in people who have no latah relative. Simons gives the following account of latah, offered by a Malaysian man, a latah himself:

> At first one is merely startled. One sees a centipede or snake or a coconut leaf falls, and one is startled. Then someone sees this happen. Later when he sees me again perhaps he'll poke me in the ribs. After a while something can happen. Take an ordinary person like Betsy here—if she's startled— whenever you see her you startle her with a poke in the ribs. After a while she'll get very frustrated! She'll say whatever comes out. If you tell her to dance, she'll dance. If you startle

her with a poke in the ribs whenever you see her, she'll do
this too [demonstrates]. That's what its like.

(Simons, 1985, p. 81).

In her study of latah, Geertz (1968) contrasted the behaviour
with the Malayo-Indonesian social norms of order, self-
control and courtesy. Taking it in its cultural context she emphasized how the behaviour of a latah contravenes and challenges the norms of the society in which it occurs. By
exhibiting behaviour which reflects an apparent lack of or-
derliness and absence of self-control and the exact opposite of
courteous behaviour, a Malayo-Indonesian can be seen as sin-
gling herself out from other members of the culture. There
could be many motivations for drawing such attention to
oneself. A common interpretation has been that marginalized
members of the society may behave in this way to protest
against how they are being treated. The person who becomes
a latah is therefore 'using' the syndrome (perhaps unconsciously) to communicate their protest.

We use the term 'culture-bound syndrome' to refer to a cluster of behaviours which occur together only in certain sociocultural contexts. We mean that the condition is not found
universally. However, an interesting feature of latah is that
apparently similar behaviours have been reported in
culturally diverse and geographically distant parts of the
world, as well as in Malaysia and Indonesia. Latah-like conditions have also been reported, albeit rarely, in Japan, South
Africa and the USA.

This appears to present us with a paradox: How can a syndrome be both 'culture bound' and found all over the world?
Two different answers to this question reflect the confusion
which can visit any practitioner confronting a condition with
which he or she is unfamiliar. The first explanation is that
latah represents a universal psychophysiological startle response (Simons, 1985): in some cultures this naturally occurring behaviour has been elaborated into stereotypical ways of

responding to being startled, among some people who are 'hyperstartlers'. Thus, according to this view all societies have 'hyperstartlers' although the behaviour associated with the startlers (e.g. swearing, jumping, hypersuggestibility) may vary across cultures. Startle behaviour may also be ignored or 'encouraged' to different extents depending on the type and amount of attention given to it.

A second explanation is to look on latah not as a universal neurophysiological event shaped by culture, but as a 'performance' relating to social norms (Kenny, 1985). This is not to deny that anybody can be startled, or that some people react more than others. This explanation says that the form which startled behaviour takes is determined not by neurophysiological events but by the norms of the society in which a person lives. How better can a Malay-Indonesian demonstrate his or her difference from other people than by contravening the social norms of order, self-control and courtesy through latah behaviour?

Thus, the second argument says that latah will coexist in different societies and cultures if the condition can perform a social function in each of those cultures. Different cultures may have different forms of latah depending on what functions are performed by it and on how the messages are best conveyed. Kenny (1985, p. 72) writes: 'The body is a symbol. Its appearance and actions point beyond itself to an inner world, but also beyond itself to a total life situation. The body expresses a state of being. . . .'

Thus, two specialists in the field of culture-bound disorders come up with two apparently similar, but actually quite different, interpretations of latah. One is that it is a universal condition, with a neurophysiological basis, shaped by different cultural contexts. The other says that it is no more a neurophysiological 'condition' than is sneezing, and its expression is purely due to the social function it can serve within a culture. The reason such an apparently small distinction is clinically important is that one may be taken as suggesting that it is a 'real' condition while the other suggests that it is a social construction and perhaps somehow less 'real'. It is to elucidate this point that we have gone into latah in some depth. Whatever explanation one favours, it should be remembered that the patient's distressing experience of latah is *their own reality*.

## WHERE DO CULTURE-BOUND SYNDROMES COME FROM?

We have considered only two culture-bound disorders in depth. Hundreds of 'culture-bound disorders' must exist. Hughes (1985) has provided a glossary of some of these. They include:

- *Bebainan*, found in Bali, where a person may suddenly break into tears and attempt to run away from their present situation. They will try to fight off anybody who tries to stop them. Ultimately they collapse with exhaustion and subsequently have no memory for these events.
- *Inarun* is a condition found among the Yoruba of Nigeria. It is characterized by weakness and burning or itching of the body, skin rashes, dimness of vision, impotence, deadness of feet and paralysis of the legs. Psychotic behaviour may also be displayed.
- *Quajimaillituq* is found among the Eskimos of the Hudson's Bay region of Canada. This is a condition of periodic hyperactivity, paranoid preoccupations, making up of new words, compulsivity and performing antisocial acts.
- *Tabacazo* is found in Chile and describes agitation, despair and aggression in association with a loss of consciousness.

When we talk of 'culture-bound disorders' it seems that we are usually referring to problems found in Asia, Africa, the Arctic regions or South America. That is, they are rarely disorders of people of European origin. While there are a large number of 'Hispanic' disorders, many of them derive from peoples indigenous to South America, rather than from the Spanish influence *per se*. Is it the case that people of European origin do not have their own 'culture-bound syndromes'? If we looked at culture-bound syndromes from a different cultural perspective, then perhaps European peoples would appear to have some bizarre behaviours too.

A glossary of syndromes bounded by 'Western' culture, or people of European origin, might include some of the following:

- *Anorexia nervosa* is usually found among adolescent females who starve themselves of food, sometimes to the point of death. As well as exhibiting extreme weight loss, amenorrhea is also common. Some sufferers also develop a distorted perception of their own body shape.
- *Type A behaviour* is most commonly exhibited by adult males as they struggle against perceived time pressure to achieve as many goals as possible. Often behaving aggressively and competitively towards others, they are also very impatient and concerned with 'deadlines'.
- *Obesity* is characterized by eating beyond the requirements of bodily functioning, resulting in excessive weight gain. This may be associated with reduced mobility, complaints of physical discomfort, disorders of mood and apparent inability to 'lose' the weight gained.
- *Agoraphobia* is a fear of leaving a restricted area, usually one's home, in case something dreadful happens. Mood disturbance and moments of panic are also common. The disorder is especially prevalent among 'housewives' who spend a lot of time inside the family home.
- *Shoplifting* is a condition where people steal goods from a shop when they are, in fact, quite capable of paying for them. This problem is usually found among financially well off, middle-aged women.
- *Exhibitionism* or *flashing* involves (usually) men dramatically displaying their genitals in public for brief periods of

time, apparently with the intention of shocking somebody close by, usually a member of the opposite sex.

In the above descriptions I have deliberately simplified and extracted particularly striking aspects of some disorders commonly found in European cultures. Each of the disorders described above is a good deal more complex than suggested by these potted descriptions. They also make a good deal more sense, given the sociocultural-cultural context, than 'foreigners' might imagine. However, I have described them in the above form as this is reminiscent of the language used to describe many (non-European) 'culture-bound syndromes'. Similarly, the language and the rationale of 'Western' drug treatments for, say, obesity may seem quite bizarre to someone from a culture where obesity does not 'exist'. They could, for instance, be forgiven for wondering why I had conducted a study evaluating the psychological correlates of an atypical beta agonist which was prescribed to increase metabolic rate with the hope of 'burning off' excess fat (MacLachlan *et al.*, 1991)! Let us explore further the culture boundness of eating disorders by considering some relevant research on anorexia nervosa.

## IS ANOREXIA NERVOSA A CULTURE-BOUND SYNDROME?

Epidemiological studies indicate that the incidence of eating disorders has increased over recent years. Most of this increase in incidence occurred in the age range 18–24. However, Khandelwal and his colleagues in Delhi have recently considered eating disorders from an Indian perspective and noted their apparent rarity in 'non-Western' cultures. While the prevalence of anorexia nervosa is undoubtedly greater in 'Western' countries, they note that some cases have in fact been reported in Iraq, Sudan, Egypt, Malaysia, Zimbabwe, Nigeria, Pakistan and India. These cases do not necessarily present the conventional symptom profile of people suffering with anorexia nervosa in the 'West', but practitioners have felt that they are similar enough to warrant the same classification.

It is intriguing to note that eating disorders are now being reported more frequently by immigrant groups in 'Western' countries. Indeed one report from England (Mumford & Whitehouse, 1988) found that there were significantly more cases of eating disorder among Asian school girls than among English school girls. Most of the Asian girls in this study were born and educated in England. This increase in the prevalence of different eating disorders—obesity, anorexia nervosa, bulimia nervosa—is not necessarily the same across different cultural groups, even within the country.

We might well ask 'Why should anorexia nervosa be a culture-bound syndrome?' Khandelwal and colleagues (1995) suggest that people in 'Western' societies are very concerned with body weight and shape and that there is aesthetic preference for thinness in women. Certain aspirations, for instance to become a dancer, are likely to coincide with an emphasis on thinness. An example of this is research showing that there is a higher risk of anorexia nervosa in those dance schools which put greater pressure on their pupils to succeed (Garner & Garfinkle, 1980). Other literature cites overdependence and at the same time hostility towards very protective parents as being characteristic of anorexia nervosa. My own work with anorexic people has impressed upon me how they may use their intake of food to demonstrate (to themselves) control over an often transitional life situation, fraught with emotional challenges and demands which they perceive to be beyond their control.

Thus from a cultural perspective the experience of anorexia nervosa among young women may be accounted for by the expectations of a 'Western' society which is ambivalent about the maturing of its daughters. These concerns are internalized by the anorexic. Yet we may be so embedded in our own culture that this is hard to grasp. Other systems of child rearing differ considerably from those in the 'West'. The very concept of adolescence would not be recognized in some other cultures, indeed it has been argued that adolescence is primarily an issue for 'Western' cultures. Elsewhere children may pass straight into the state of 'adulthood' often following their initiation at the age of 13 or 14. They assume the roles and responsibilities of adults immediately. From their perspective the slow 'letting go' of the parents and the 'building in maturity' of the youngster are no doubt curious.

If anorexia nervosa is a disorder of 'Western' maturation then it is hardly surprising that people in other cultures don't (have the need to) experience it. However, when members of 'foreign' cultural groups have become part of 'Western' societies, then such disorders do become more common. They have a reason for being. Indeed their higher rates may in some cases represent their use as an expression of the dynamics between different cultures. For instance, an Asian girl who develops an 'English disorder' could be interpreted as demonstrating her identity with England and rejecting her Asian ancestry. In this way 'culture-bound disorders' may be used to 'manage' the demanding interplay between different cultural traditions. If this is indeed true then further research might find an important relationship between different patterns of acculturation and the sort of disorders which people develop.

We have not fully answered the question of whether anorexia nervosa is a culture-bound disorder or not. In one sense it appears to be: it is generally found in 'Western' peoples or minority cultural groups who have come to live in the 'West'. Yet in some forms, albeit rarely, it is found elsewhere. You may recall that this is a rather similar situation to that with 'latah'. It seems to be the case that certain conditions are generally 'culture bound' but occasionally may also occur outside of that culture.

A classic adage in architecture is that 'form should not give way to function'. That is to say, the way something looks should not be primarily determined by what it is to do. The aesthetic value of an object is important, not just its use. This distinction between form and function may be useful for understanding 'culture-bound syndromes'. The 'form', in this context, is the way in which a problem is presented—self-starvation, stealing unwanted goods, fearing genital shrinkage, reacting with extreme startle. The 'function', again in our context, refers to what the event can achieve within the cultural context where it is present. Thus restating this architectural adage one might say that 'form serves function'. In that different cultures requires things to be done in different ways to achieve the same ends, form may well have to give way to function. Indeed it is often where form fails to give way to (our understanding of how things) function, that we define a condition as being bound outside our own culture.

It has been argued that all disorder is related to cultural factors and that, by implication, some cultures 'encourage' some sorts of disorder while other cultures 'encourage' different forms of disorder. Weisz *et al.* (1987) set out to examine how the cultures children were brought up in were related to the sorts of disorders children develop. They considered two alternative models. The *suppression–facilitation* model suggests that cultures facilitate the development of some behaviours through rewarding children for them, and suppress the development of other behaviours through punishing them, or failing to reward them. This model suggests that the problem behaviours presented by children in the clinic will be similar to those behaviours which are culturally encouraged, except that they will be performed to an excessive extent. An alternative model, the *adult distress threshold* model, suggests that problem behaviours presented in the clinic will, in contrast, be those which are discouraged, because parents are less tolerant of them.

Weisz *et al.* compared children referred to clinics in Thailand and the USA. Weisz *et al.* characterized the Thai culture as emphasizing peacefulness and non-aggression, and the importance of being polite, modest and deferential towards others. Parents in Thai culture were seen as being intolerant of under-controlled, aggressive and disrespectful behaviour. Consistent with the suppression–facilitation model they found that Thai children referred to clinics tended to exhibit over-controlled behaviours, such as, inhibition, anxiety and fearfulness. Weisz *et al.* characterized USA culture as being more tolerant of aggressiveness, encouraging self-expression, independence and assertiveness. Once again, consistent with the suppression–facilitation model, they found that children referred to clinics in the USA tended to exhibit under-controlled behaviours, such as aggression, impulsivity and distractibility. This research therefore suggests the very important point that culture influences the exhibition of disorder, not only through symbolism, but also through behavioural mechanisms.

## ANALYSING HEALTH THROUGH CULTURE

Despite the seemingly vast array of forms of suffering which are found across different cultures, there are in fact a finite number of ways in which we can express our distress. Classification of different forms of suffering is an attempt to simplify their complexity. Yet an appropriate classification may give great conceptual insights to the nature of suffering. It is argued here that the term 'culture-bound syndrome' is something of a misnomer. Presumably all suffering is to some extent influenced by the context in which it occurs. However, the use of the term 'culture-bound syndrome' could be taken to suggest that some forms of suffering are influenced by culture while others are not. The value of the 'culture-bound' approach is that it turns our attention to the contextual factors which may play a role in human suffering. We should embrace the benefits of this approach by applying it to all types of suffering, whatever their cultural or geographical origins (Hughes, 1985).

Figure 3.1 shows four levels through which culture may influence suffering. Firstly there is the *causal* level—that is, the

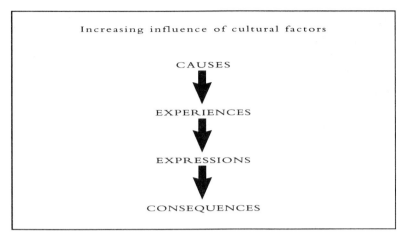

**Figure 3.1:** Levels of suffering

agent responsible for bringing about the suffering. Such causal factors could include infection, bewitchment, reinforcement and stress, to mention just a few. Clearly people's beliefs about the cause of a problem will be influenced by socio-cultural factors. The practitioner must also appreciate the extent to which their own beliefs are shaped by such factors. Whatever working hypotheses are used to describe the cause of suffering, the clinician needs to appreciate the extent to which different hypothetical causes are influenced by culture.

The next level at which culture may influence suffering is at the level of *experience*. Thus the way in which we know that we are suffering may be influenced by our physical environment and the people around us. This level is concerned with the form of suffering. A Chinese person may suffer from stress through somatization—developing aches and pains—while a German person might suffer from stress through cognitization—focusing on the negative aspects of their life and having a poor self-concept. Here somatization and cognitization may be different forms of suffering, brought on by similar circumstances. It is through the experience of physical aches and pains or through the experience of negativity and poor self-concept that a person knows he or she is suffering.

The next level is concerned with the *expression* of suffering. This can be taken at two levels. One level is the private level which constitutes the content of the suffering: which parts of the body have the aches and pains, or what are the negative thoughts actually about? The other level is more public and is to do with how such suffering is displayed. One display of negativity might be to withdraw into a corner in order to avoid contact with other people. Another form of negativity could be to tell other people about all the problems and pessimism which you harbour. As well as individual differences, cultures also differ in their norms for the expression of suffering. In some cultures people cry openly and hysterically at funerals while in others people are very stoical.

Finally, the fourth level concerns the *consequences* of suffering. The consequences of suffering may be very different in different cultures. At one extreme, recall the bride who people believed was undergoing a koro attack, and their subsequent efforts to 'rescue' her and alleviate her suffering. At the other extreme must be the 'bystander apathy' effect— a social psychological phenomenon often exhibited in urban areas of the 'West', where a person who is obviously suffering (perhaps even being 'mugged') is ignored by those close by them. More generally the expression of suffering may attract sympathy, pity, help, frustration, anger and so on. Each of these reactions will be influenced by the socio-cultural meaning of suffering.

Perhaps the key question to understanding a culture's influence on welfare and suffering is this: 'Is suffering a product of the culture or does it exist independently of it?'. Volumes of research literature attest to the important impact which culture has in shaping the causes, experiences, expressions and consequences of suffering. Yet it is also undeniable that some suffering is beyond the bounds of culture. For instance, the contraction of meningitis in an infant will result in predictable symptoms whether it occurs in Dublin, Delhi or Durban. A gunshot wound in the thigh will have certain similar features whether it occurs in Belfast, Berlin or Bombay. One could, of course, argue that certain forms of suffering (for instance, gunshot wounds) are found more frequently in some places than in others, and relate this to environmental and/or cultural factors. This is a valid argument but beyond the scope of the present chapter.

From the perspective of the clinician, it is important to recognize that some forms of suffering will not be attributable to culture, at least at the objective causal level. Subjective causes are obviously related to culture. I would suggest that as one moves along the chain *cause–experience–expression–consequence*, at each step culture makes a progressively greater contribution to the person's suffering. This sequence of suffering is therefore a useful way for the clinician to think about the interplay between culture and suffering.

## GUIDELINES FOR PROFESSIONAL PRACTICE

1. A person's beliefs about illness may reflect social myths and social desirability within their culture. The social functions of illness can be expected to influence not only the beliefs of the lay public but also the beliefs of health professionals. Clinicians should consider what social functions are served by their own way of working.
2. Although the idea of 'culture-bound syndromes' is well established it may lead clinicians to assume that most syndromes ('non-culture-bound syndromes') are uninfluenced by the culture they are expressed in. This would be a dangerous assumption and often reflects the erroneous belief that 'our own' syndromes are not influenced by our culture. All syndromes are, at least to some extent, influenced by their cultural context. So, too, is the way in which clinicians respond to them.
3. The exotic nature of many 'culture-bound syndromes' can deflect the clinician from analysing their social meaning and function. The clinician should avoid discounting ap-

parently bizarre conditions and investigate them in terms of their order and function.

4. The problems with which an individual presents may be a reflection of more than their own state of well-being; they may, for instance, also reflect anxiety within their wider community. In such a case the individual who presents the problem may be a social scapegoat, as in the case of koro. It is therefore important to look beyond the client to his or her community and culture.

5. Some theorists see the human body as a symbol which can be moulded by culture into different types of suffering. Other theorists believe that there are some basic and universal bodily experiences and that the extent to which, and manner by which, these experiences are expressed is influenced by culture. The important point for the clinicians to remember is that neither of these accounts diminishes the genuineness of their client's experience of suffering.

6. 'Culture-bound syndromes' do not come from somewhere else. Many European and North American conditions are equally influenced by culture. Understanding the cultural construction of disorders common to one's own people can be difficult because it calls for the clinician to fight against his or her ethnocentricity and see their own culture as one among many.

7. Sometimes indigenous 'culture-bound syndromes' can be seen to increase in incidence among immigrant groups. This should not be taken as indicating that a syndrome is not 'culture bound' but may instead reflect the acculturation of the immigrant group, such that some of its members express their problems though local cultural idioms.

8. Suffering can be described at the levels of 'causes', 'experiences', 'expressions' and 'consequences'. On average, culture will have a progressively greater influence the further down this chain one travels.

# 4

# CULTURE AND MENTAL HEALTH

This chapter builds on our review of culture-bound syndromes in Chapter 3. We consider in detail the issue of depression and to what extent, and in what form, it may be said to occur in different parts of the world. The complexities of understanding depression across cultures can be taken as a model for analysing many different mental problems. We also consider personality disorders in the context of minority cultural groups. This is an especially interesting and difficult area because personality disorders are often classified in relation to the social norms to which a person fails to adhere. People who are not socialized in a culture's norms may therefore be at greater risk of being misclassified as exhibiting a personality disorder. Migrant groups encounter a broad range of stressors as part of their transition. These may lead to mental problems or to physical problems, or both. Indeed the dichotomy I have drawn between mental and physical health is a culturally based one and in many cultures would be taken as quite arbitrary. This distinction is made only for the convenience of dividing our discussion into chapters. The final section of this chapter considers how stress can cause physical problems and this is then developed further in Chapter 5.

## WAYS OF STUDYING MENTAL HEALTH ACROSS CULTURES

Cultural differences in mental health have been studied in a number of different ways. First there was the *comparative* approach which compared the incidence and prevalence of mental problems in different parts of the world. Generally this research sought to establish the extent to which mental health problems occurring in the 'West' also occurred elsewhere. The prevalence and incidence of 'Western' disorders were therefore compared across geographically distinct cultures. The research question motivating such studies was: 'Do different cultures show the same rate of (Western) mental disorders?' Another important research question arising out of this comparative approach was: 'Do different cultures give rise to different mental disorders?'. In other words, are there disorders which are particular to some cultures and not to others?

A second approach developed with the empowerment of minority culture groups which had either established a presence in a foreign country, or established a voice in their own country, despite it being governed by 'foreigners'. An example of the former is Afro-Caribbeans establishing a significant community in London by the late 1960s. An example of the latter is the contemporary empowerment of Canada's indigenous peoples in establishing 'First Nations' rights. This can be described as the *cultural minority* approach because the people of interest were usually minority culture groups acting within a different sociocultural context to the majority culture group(s). The main research question here was: 'Do cultural minorities have particular mental health problems distinct from the majority society in which they are living?'

A third approach to the study of mental disorders across cultures is the *transitional* approach. The focus here is with people who have left their home country or region to relocate elsewhere. This may be on a temporary or permanent basis, as with sojourners or immigrants. It may also be voluntarily or forced, immigrants usually being an example of voluntary transition, while refugees are an example of forced transition. The major research question in this approach has been: 'How are the stresses of transition and acculturation dealt with and manifested?'

The above classification is neither comprehensive nor mutually exclusive. Furthermore, research from the comparative, cultural minority and transitional perspectives, may all be brought to bear on similar issues. The different approaches have grown out of the historical and political contexts in which cross-cultural research has been conducted. The ethnocentrism of the comparative approach reflects many of the colonial values of the late nineteenth and early twentieth century: 'How similar to us are these people?' The cultural minority approach expresses a concern for how (well) society can cope with subcultures which often have little democratic, economic or professional influence within the majority culture. The Los Angeles riots of 1994 were a recent and dramatic foci for this problem. For the transitional approach, the tides of war refugees are an equally dramatic example of the political spasms of a world in complex disorder. In 1997, Hong Kong will revert to the jurisdiction of China, after 99 years of British rule. The people of Hong Kong may have to adapt, not only to a change of government or nationality, but also to different cultural expectations, economic realities and political ethos. Without going to war, hopefully, and without relocating, the citizens of Hong Kong have become 'transitional people', in the sense of adapting to an important change in their life situation.

These cultural complexities are no longer beyond the ken of the average person. They are beamed into our sitting rooms so that we are presented with the anguish, the fear, the suffering of people struggling to come to terms with the meaning of their existence. Cross-cultural services for mental health have never been more important, or as inescapable, as they are now. In this chapter we explore each of the three

approaches to studying culture and mental health. We de-
bunk some old myths, highlight some recent innovations in
research and provide the clinician with an informed context in
which to (co-)operate.

## COMPARATIVE MENTAL HEALTH

It would be possible to give a sort of epidemiological audit of
the incidence and prevalence of a spectrum of mental disorders across different cultures. Such information might well
be useful if it truly reflected the health service needs of different cultural groups. However, one difficulty here is that
epidemiological data is inevitably generated from a particular perspective, a particular way of classifying mental well-
being and mental disorder. Nowhere are the intricacies of
this problem more clearly demonstrated than in the case of
depression. We will therefore use the case of depression to
explore the complexities of comparing mental health across
cultures.

Depression has been described as 'the common cold of psychopathology'. Indeed it is a relatively common form of distress experienced to some extent by most 'Westernized'
people at some time in their life. Statistical estimates vary;
however, on average, 'Western' studies have found a prevalence (the percentage of people who experience the condition
at a given time) of between 9 and 20 per cent for significant
symptoms of depression (e.g. Boyd & Weissman, 1981), and
that women are twice as likely to experience clinical depression compared with men. Depression also appears to be more
frequently identified now than it was 50 years ago, perhaps
up to 10 times more. This increase in depression in the 'West'
may be accounted for by factors such as the decline of religion, changes in community environments, more frequent
uprooting of individuals and families from one locale to another, disintegration of family structures and the increased
social isolation of some people (Sartorius, 1989).

Most of the existing statistics on depression refer only to those who experience depression to a severity sufficient to warrant a diagnosis of clinical depression. The depressed mood which most people experience is, thankfully, not of great severity and lacking many of the other features which define depression of clinical severity. So what are the characteristics of depression of clinical severity?

The two most prominent 'Western' systems of classification have an inherent assumption that their criteria may be globally applied to give valid and reliable diagnoses. These two classification systems are DSM-IV (*Diagnostic and Statistical Manual* of the American Psychiatric Association, fourth edition) and ICD-10 (*International Classification of Diseases*, tenth edition). For many conditions there is very little difference between the criteria used in each of the two systems. Since depression is one of the conditions on which there seems to be strong convergence, let us look at only one of these systems for a definition of depression.

DSM-IV recognizes several different sorts (or subtypes) of depression including dysthymia, adjustment disorder with depressed mood, major depressive disorder, cyclothymia, bipolar disorder (manic-depression) and mood disorders associated with other primary problems such as substance abuse or a serious medical condition. Major depressive disorder is the condition I want to concentrate on because more cross-cultural research has been done on this type than any other type of psychological/psychiatric disorder. According to DSM-IV an episode of major depressive disorder ('depression' from here on) is said to exist when a person experiences either a markedly depressed mood or a marked loss of interest in pleasurable activities for most of the day, every day, for at least two weeks. In addition to this, the person must simultaneously experience at least four or more of the following symptoms: significant weight loss (when not dieting) or weight gain, or a decrease or increase in appetite; undersleeping (insomnia) or oversleeping (hypersomnia); slowing down (psychomotor retardation) or speeding up (psychomotor agitation) of mental and physical activity; fatigue or loss of energy; feelings of worthlessness or excessive or inappropriate guilt; diminished ability to think or concentrate or indecisiveness; and recurrent thoughts of death or suicide.

Kleinman (1980) has suggested that the way in which people experience distress (such as depression) varies across cultures and at different times within the same culture. He uses the word 'illness' (as many people do) to refer to a person's experience of a disease. Most of the diseases which affect the body are not observed at their source of action. Instead it is the consequences of the disease's actions—the rash, the limp, the lethargy, etc.—which is observed. This 'illness behaviour' includes our physical and mental responses to a disease. For the moment, it is the psychological component of this response to disease which is of interest to us. A key point in Kleinman's argument is that illness behaviour is the result of an underlying disease process and that this disease process may be expressed in different forms of illness behaviour.

Now at first inspection this distinction between disease and illness seems a very useful one because it helps us to account for the admittedly vast array of symptoms associated with a diagnosis (of the disease) depression. According to the diagnostic criteria described above, two people may be depressed, but their experience of being depressed may be quite different. For instance, one person may have depressed mood, weight loss, poor appetite, difficulty sleeping and behave in a very slow and withdrawn manner. Another person, with the same diagnosis, may not experience depressed mood at all. Instead they may show a loss of interest or pleasure in many different activities, gain weight, feel constantly hungry, oversleep and appear very agitated. However, according to the DSM-IV criteria their very different 'illness behaviours' are explained by the presence of the same underlying disease process. This understanding of depression has its critics, and I'm one of them. In psychological terms it is better to think of people as suffering *with* (or through) what they are experiencing—early morning wakening, low self-esteem, depressed mood and so on—not *from* something else. In terms of DSM-IV and ICD-10, however, people are usually suffering from something else, an underlying disease entity, not from their immediate experience.

The experience of depression within an individual can vary over time (commonly referred to as the disease course) and, as already noted, it can vary between individuals of the same culture (commonly referred to as a disease syndrome). Kleinman's suggestion that depression can also vary across cultures and across different historical epochs is quite consistent with a biological view of depression. He has also studied a condition known as neurasthenia. This condition, commonly reported in China, is characterized by a lack of energy and physical complaints such as a sore stomach. Kleinman has suggested that while depression and neurasthenia are different illness experiences, they are both products of the same underlying disease processes—depression. In other words, neurasthenia is the Chinese version of the 'Western' depression.

Shweder (1991) suggests that this interpretation 'privileges' a biological understanding of how depression occurs. He points out a range of factors which can theoretically cause depression, including biological ones. Table 4.1 illustrates the different factors in what he calls biomedical, moral, sociopolitical, interpersonal and psychological 'causal ontologies'. Now things become complicated. Kleinman believes that the ultimate cause of depression and neurasthenia is the same. This ultimate cause concerns the experiences of defeat, loss, vexation and oppression by local hierarchies of power. Such 'sociopolitical' experiences produce a biological disease process. However, the way in which this disease is expressed is influenced by the culture within which one lives.

Some forms of suffering—because they can be understood to provide a message, a communication—are more acceptable

**Table 4.1:** Different types of causes for depression

| Domain | Factors |
|--------|---------|
| Biomedical | Organ pathology<br>Physiological impairment<br>Hormone imbalance |
| Moral | Transgression<br>Sin<br>Karma |
| Sociopolitical | Oppression<br>Injustice<br>Loss |
| Interpersonal | Envy<br>Hatred<br>Sorcery |
| Psychological | Anger<br>Desire<br>Intrapsychic conflict<br>Defence |

Based on Shweder (1991).

than others. In North America, for instance, there is a great emphasis on individualism, competitiveness, slogging it out in the market place, achieving, personal growth, realizing one's own (amazing!) potential, and so on. There is also a great emphasis on 'letting it out', on the right of the individual to openly express what she or he feels. This allows for the expression of depression as a demonstration of the individual's disillusionment with not 'succeeding'. On the other hand, in China, or so it can be argued, depression is not the 'right' form of suffering. In China demoralization and hopelessness may be stigmatized as losing faith in the political ideals of 'the system'. Such a public display of disengagement is not welcome. Instead a variety of symptoms consistent with fatigue, with being physically run down, with being exhausted by the pressures of work, may be seen as an acceptable reason for failure.

In summary then, Kleinman is suggesting that depression and neurasthenia have similar sociopolitical origins which produce a similar biological disease process, which expresses itself differently in North America and China because the different cultural conditions favour different forms of expression. Once again this seems to be a perfectly reasonable argument. However, Shweder makes the perfectly reasonable criticism that there is no need to say that the Chinese's neurasthenia is somatized depression. We might just as well say that North American depression is emotionalized neurasthenia and that neurasthenia is the underlying disease process, not depression. However, Shweder questions the value of talking about disease processes at all. For him, the concepts of 'illness' and 'disease' do not add any value to our understanding of the relationship between neurasthenia and depression. While these two conditions may have similar origins in sociopolitical adversity, we are able to distinguish between the two forms of suffering. If there is, therefore, no need to think in terms of a biological 'middle man', then there is no need for either neurasthenia or depression to be the primary disorder.

How acceptable you find this conclusion will no doubt depend on your own professional (= subcultural) training. However, you may still ask, 'Does it really matter?' Well, yes it does. If Mr Lim presents symptoms of neurasthenia in my Dublin clinic and I interpret him as 'really suffering from depression', then my interpretation of his condition may be radically different from his experience of his condition. Turn it the other way round: if you go to the doctor in Beijing and she tells you that you're not really depressed as such, but that you are really suffering from stomach problems, then you are unlikely to feel understood (and you may wonder if you took a wrong turn somewhere along the hospital's maze of corridors!).

Does it really matter in terms of treatment? This may well depend on your method of treatment. If it involves

prescribing 'antidepressant' medication then (paradoxically)
Mr Lim may be happier having that for his neurasthenia than
many 'Westerners' would be having it for their depression.
Incidentally, even if the same medication is effective for both
conditions, it doesn't necessarily mean that they share the
same cause (I may take an Aspirin for a headache and a tooth-
ache, but it doesn't mean that I have a hole in my cranium
corresponding to the hole in my tooth). Returning to Mr Lim's
neurasthenia, if I think he is 'really depressed' and try out
Beck's cognitive therapy on a man who doesn't report any
cognitive symptoms of depression, then I may only worsen
his problems. The reason for the distinction between neurasthenia and depression being so important, and for the
practitioner to acknowledge it, is that in doing so we are
acknowledging the person's experience of their own suffering. We are not imposing our culturally myopic perspective
on another human being in order to treat a problem we know
about, even if it is not the problem they are suffering from. In
short, we are being clinically practical, not hegemonically
theoretical.

## Diagnosis

But again, does it really matter if they are so similar in any
case? Yes is does, because they are not necessarily so similar
after all. If DSM criteria are used to classify Chinese neu-
rasthenics, a good proportion of them do not fulfil the criteria for depression. Also, a good proportion of North
American depressives do not fulfil the Chinese criteria for
neurasthenia. Thus their distressing experiences are different. We can only join them together by assuming a biological syndromal model of depression, world wide. This idea is
that everybody suffers from the same things that we do,
except that they express it differently. The idea that neurasthenia is 'masked depression', subsumes the experience
of somatization under depression. It gives primary importance to the depression.

This assumed primacy of depression over somatic symptoms has recently been explored in Banglagore, India. Mitchell Weiss and colleagues (1995) sought to explore the relationship between depressive, anxious and somatoform experiences, not only from the 'Western' diagnostic perspective of the DSM classification systems, but also from the perspective of individuals' own illness experiences. Their study used established structured interview schedules to glean both types of information from their interviewees who were all first-time presenting psychiatric out-patients attending a clinic in Banglagore. When the same 'symptom' presentation was interpreted by the patient and by the DSM system, generally patients preferred to describe their problems in terms of somatic symptoms while the DSM system described them in terms of depression.

It is important to point out that the experience of somatic symptoms is also common in European and North American contexts. Indeed 'Somatization Disorder' is a recognized diagnostic category in the DSM classification system. Such a diagnosis is made when people report somatic distress without any evidence of organic cause. A recent study of somatization in primary care settings in Spain reported that almost 10 per cent of people presenting a new episode of illness to a primary care clinic, and approximately one-third of people who presented psychological problems which were severe enough to be classified as 'psychiatric cases', fulfilled the criteria for somatization (Lobo *et al.*, 1996; Garcia-Campayo *et al.*, 1996). Table 4.2 gives the frequency of somatic symptoms most commonly reported in 147 Spanish somatizers. Back ache, dizziness and pains in extremities were cited by over 60 per cent of somatizers. The table illustrates a wide range of somatic distress, including problems which may not often be associated with this diagnosis, such as diarrhoea, vomiting, trouble walking and urinary retention. The majority of these somatizing patients fulfilled the criteria for DSM-IV diagnoses of depression or anxiety.

The Spanish investigators subdivided their 'psychiatric' sample into 'somatizers' (described above) and 'psychologizers',

**Table 4.2:** Most frequent somatic symptoms in Spanish somatizers ($n$ = 147)

| Somatic symptoms | Percentage |
|---|---|
| Back pain | 71.4 |
| Dizziness | 65.3 |
| Pain in extremities | 60.5 |
| Bloating (gassy) | 52.3 |
| Shortness of breath | 50.3 |
| Palpitations | 49.6 |
| Joint pain | 45.5 |
| Chest pain | 44.2 |
| Nausea (other than motion sickness) | 43.5 |
| Amnesia | 39.4 |
| Abdominal pain | 37.4 |
| Intolerance of different foods | 24.4 |
| Diarrhoea | 23.1 |
| Difficulty swallowing | 21.7 |
| Painful menstruation* | 21.4 |
| Blurred vision | 20.4 |
| Paralysis or muscle weakness | 20.4 |
| Excessive menstrual bleeding* | 18.6 |
| Sexual indifference | 17.6 |
| Trouble walking | 17.0 |
| Irregular menstrual periods* | 15.8 |
| Vomiting (other than during pregnancy) | 14.9 |
| Pain during urination | 14.2 |
| Loss of voice | 11.5 |
| Urinary retention | 10.2 |

* Only in women.
Reproduced from Lobo *et al.* (1966) with permission.

of whom there were 46. Thus three times as many 'psychiatric' patients were rated as 'somatizers' rather than 'psychologizers'. The most frequent diagnosis made for 'somatizers' was Generalized Anxiety Disorder, while for 'psychologizers' it was Major Depression. Table 4.3 shows the DSM-IV diagnoses given to the whole sample. As can be seen here there is substantial overlap between these two groups and the

**Table 4.3:** DSM–IV diagnosis in Spanish somatizers and psychologizers

| Diagnosis (DSM–IV) | Somatizers | | Psychologizers | |
|---|---|---|---|---|
| | $n = 147$ (%) | | $n = 46$ (%) | |
| Generalized anxiety disorder | 32 | (21.7) | 12 | (26.0) |
| Depressive disorder NOS | 23 | (15.6) | 11 | (23.9) |
| Major depression | 22 | (14.9) | 13 | (28.2) |
| Dysthymia | 21 | (14.2) | 2 | (4.3) |
| Somatization disorder | 14 | (9.5) | | – |
| Adjustment disorder | 12 | (8.1) | 5 | (10.8) |
| Undifferentiated somatoform disorder | 7 | (4.7) | | – |
| Panic disorder/agoraphobia | 3 | (2.0) | | – |
| Others | 13 | (8.8) | 3 | (6.5) |

NOS = not otherwise stated.
Reproduced from Garcia-Campayo et al. (1996) with permission.

diagnostic categories used. The most dramatic contrast is for the diagnosis of dysthymia, which refers to a chronic (at least two years) although less severe form of depression than major depressive disorder. In the dysthymic category there was a ratio of 10 : 1 between 'somatizers' and 'psychologizers'.

Such results, and many others like them, illustrate the complexity of understanding and categorizing the distress which people present to practitioners. Indeed we do not need to go to China to find that many people presenting physical problems receive a diagnosis of depression. We do not need to go to China to ask about similarities and differences between the underlying nature of presenting complaints. These dilemmas are on our own doorstep. As so often is the case in cross-cultural psychology, comparisons between cultures can also sharpen the focus on one's own culture. Our own cultural assumptions often blind us to our own complexities. This is hardly surprising since assumptions are often simplifications to make the world more manageable. In short, we do not only stereotype other cultures, we also stereotype our own. Wherever you come from, your people are quite complicated too!

In the 'West', people are so versed in the notion of psycho-somatic problems (where the psychic is primary and the soma secondary) that even contemplating the somatopsychic (where the soma is primary and the psychic secondary), is hard going. As a psychologist, even writing the very word 'somatopsychic' makes me feel awkward. Furthermore, although we use diagnostic systems to try to simplify the phenomena we encounter, these systems are so much a product of our cultural and professional (subcultural) thinking, that they may veil the true experience of an individual's suffering. Weiss *et al.* (1995), commenting on their results, write:

> These limitations of the diagnostic system identified here appear to reside more with the professional construction of categories than with the inability of patients and professionals to comprehend each other's concepts of distress and disorder. . . . Personal meanings and other aspects of phenomenological and subjective experience should be incorporated into psychiatric evaluation and practice . . . facilitating an empathic clinical alliance and enabling a therapist to work with patients' beliefs over the course of treatment. . . .

Thus whatever the presenting complaint, the belief system of the person who 'owns' the complaint has to be the medium for working through. The context of the presentation—not an abstracted diagnostic system—is what gives the complaint meaning. Without taking the context into account, clinically we can misinterpret the meaning of somatic complaints to be the 'masked' presence of cognitive distortions, low self-esteem, low mood and so on.

## Lessons from the developing world

Psychology as a discipline is strongly associated with Euro-American thinking. However, psychology as an activity exists in all human beings and, indeed, even in the so-called 'lower' species of animals. Psychology is a universal activity. Unless we were all to some extent psychologists, communication would be impossible. There can be little doubt that, for instance, Asian, African and South American psychologies are every bit as complex and sophisticated as the (false) amalgam of Euro-American psychology. While alternative psychologies do have a voice in 'Western' societies, they tend to be marginalized. Most of the 'psychological traffic' is in one direction, from Europe and America outwards towards the less industrialized ('developing') countries. This has resulted in a degree of psychological colonization, where 'foreign' peoples are encouraged to think that the Euro-American way of thinking is the right way of thinking. Such a position is an affront to the thousands of indigenous psychologies which have existed for generations. It is to be hoped that, apart from nurturing aspects of our own psychologies, each of us can also learn something from different ways of being in the world. Within this spirit Schumaker (1996) has recently set out to explore some of the lessons which the less 'developed' countries may have for the more 'developed' countries, especially regarding an understanding of depression. As will be seen, there is much to learn.

Two of the most prominent models of psychopathology in the 'West'—the cognitively based psychological model and the biologically based medical model—both locate the origin of psychopathology in the individual. In essence, because these individualist models do not take cultural factors into account, they assume universalism: that every individual, given appropriate cognitive/biological conditions, is at risk of becoming depressed. We have already explored the complexities of understanding the possibility of depression being expressed in different ways in different cultures. However, Schumaker

(1996) explores the intriguing possibility of cultures which are free of all symptoms associated with depression, including somatic symptoms.

The Kaluli of New Guinea have no word in their language for 'depression' and do not recognize the 'Western' description of depression. Is it possible that some aspects of Kaluli culture—of their way of living in the world—protect against depression? One striking feature of the culture appears to be a propensity to get angry, with social displays of anger being encouraged and used to rank the status of a person. Among the Kaluli it's good to get angry because it stimulates attempts at compensation. According to the principle of social reciprocity, a person who is angered deserves to have things 'made up' to them. Being angry is therefore a good way to get what you want. It does not induce antagonism or grudges. The Kaluli reaction to anger is therefore significantly different from that in 'Western' cultures.

A psychoanalytic explanation of depression is that it represents the results of anger towards another person being turned inwards, on the self. So, for example, the loss of a loved one may produce not only feelings of great sadness but also feelings of desertion. Usually it is not acceptable to be angry at the person who has died, and so rather than displaying this anger, and because it cannot simply disappear, it is turned against the self, perhaps being experienced as guilt and self-depreciation leading to depression. Might it then be the case that the Kaluli do not get depressed because they live in a society in which anger need not be turned inwards upon the self, but can instead be projected outwards in a socially sanctioned display? Indeed this might be the case. Often such conclusions are drawn on comparisons between 'Western' culture and another culture. However, spreading the cross-cultural comparison net wider proves to be even more informative.

The Toraja of Indonesia is another culture in which depression does not appear to be experienced. However, among the

Toraja it is not good to display anger. Anger is shameful and dangerous and may result in punishment from supernatural forces, resulting in physical and mental suffering. It is not just the social expression of anger which is to be avoided, one should not feel anger, even if it goes unexpressed. This then seems to eliminate the expression of anger as the sole responsible cause for the Kaluli's freedom from depression. Schumaker argues that what distinguishes how many 'Western' cultures deal with anger from how Toraja culture deals with it, is that while anger is clearly undesirable in Toraja culture it is not relegated to the 'social unconscious' as it is in many 'Western' cultures. In other words, the Toraja see anger as an expected reaction to certain situations and as an issue to be dealt with, to be worked through. 'Western' societies, it is argued, do not afford the same inevitability to anger. Rather than individuals being encouraged to deal with angry feelings they are expected not to work through them but to tuck them away, to hide them, to banish them. It is this banishment of emotion from social discourse which constitutes the anger being turned inwards which may be associated with depression in many 'Western' cultures.

The apparent non-occurrence of depression in the Kaluli and Toraja and countless other cultures, challenges assumptions about the universality of this form of suffering. It is particularly a problem for the biological model which assumes that a particular disease process will inevitably result in a corresponding disease experience. It is less of a problem for psychosocial models of depression because these models do at least allow for the malleability of psychosocial processes. However, there is still a problem here. Quite understandably, Schumaker, writing from Australia, attempts to understand the occurrence or non-occurrence of depression across diverse cultures by reference to the psychoanalytic formulation of anger turned inwards. While this is clearly a 'Western' concept it is also true that we can only work on problems for which we have the tools available. Schumaker should not be criticized for putting these tools (concepts) to use in unravelling this intriguing mystery of why some cultures ex-perience 'depression' and others do not.

It will be very difficult to identify one factor, such as the internalization of anger, which accounts for the varied experi-ence of depression across cultures. Cultures are 'package holi-days' for life. There is a whole lot thrown in and these many factors will probably interact in unique ways in their different social and geographical contexts. This should not stop us searching for factors salient to human health and welfare, but it should encourage us to broaden our net to multifactorial causes. For the practitioner working across cultures, some understanding of the process of interaction between variables is going to be a more achievable goal than identifying the salient content of causation across many cultures. Depression has exemplified many of the complexities of understanding mental distress in the context of culture. We now turn to consider the relationship between cultural minorities and mental health.

## CULTURAL MINORITY MENTAL HEALTH

### Group densities

In recent years a great deal of concern has been expressed about the high rates of mental disorder in cultural (or ethnic) minority groups. In both studies of admission to psychiatric facilities and in studies of 'psychiatric case' prevalence in the community, cultural minorities have been over-represented in comparison to members of their host culture. Culture is only one of a range of factors which have been associated with a higher rate of mental disturbance. Over the last 30 years Brown and his colleagues, working mostly in London, have illuminated a range of 'risk factors' for mental disorder. These factors include social class, employment status, gender, social support, personal history and situational demands. For in-stance, in their classic book *The Social Origins of Depression*

(1978), Brown and Harris reported that women who had experienced the death of their own mother before the age of 11, who did not have an intimate relationship with their partner, and who were at home caring for three or more young children were more likely to develop depression of clinical severity than women who had not experienced these psychosocial stressors. Research of this sort drew attention to the neglected influence which social contexts can have on mental functioning.

This sort of analysis also encouraged researchers to identify sociocultural factors which may be responsible for the observed high rates of mental disorder in cultural minority groups. However, membership of a cultural minority group is not simply a cultural phenomenon. It is often the case that the most socially and economically disadvantaged groups in a society are the groups which have most recently immigrated into the country. Such groups are often expected to join the 'bottom of the pile' and to work their way up—something like an 'acculturation apprenticeship', where it is expected that you will have it rough to begin with, but that, in time (with effort) things will come good in the end. The multiplicity of social and economic factors implicated in cultural minority status has made it difficult to identify the extent to which being a member of a minority culture group is, in and of itself, a stress factor related to mental disorder. However, a recent analysis of cultural minority group densities offers the clinician a social psychological framework for understanding mental health in the community.

Halpern (1993) has shown how previously contradictory research can be accommodated within his theory of group densities. First of all, let's consider some of the contradictory research findings. American blacks tend, as an overall group, to have higher first admission rates to psychiatric facilities than do American whites, as an overall group. However, if we look within each of these groups something very interesting becomes apparent. The whites with the highest rates of

admission are those who live in primarily black areas. Previously this finding had been explained in terms of 'social
drift': that poorer white people, who could only afford to live
in the poorer areas of cities, experienced the social and economic difficulties of living in poor areas and that this resulted
in increased social stress, which produced higher than average (for white people) rates of admission. These white people
had 'drifted' down to the lowest socioeconomic sector of
society, where, because of the immigrant history of the USA,
they were now in the minority. An alternative, but related
explanation was in terms of 'selection': other things being
equal, the poor and/or people from minority cultures were
more likely to be admitted to a psychiatric institution because
clinicians were more willing to admit them than they were to
admit middle-class or more 'successful' people.

However, within the black group the highest rates of admission were among those people who lived in areas where
blacks were in the minority. Thus blacks living in middle-
class white American 'good' areas had higher admission rates
than blacks living in the more deprived areas. Given the superior services and facilities enjoyed by predominantly white
communities in the USA, downward 'social drift' could obviously not be the explanation for their higher morbidity relative to their white co-residents. Nor could 'selection' be the
explanation, for why would middle-class blacks be 'selected'
for admission over poorer black people.

Further research on other cultural groups has shown that the
larger the number of people in a minority cultural group living within a given area, the lower the psychiatric admission
rate for minority cultural group members in that area. This
suggests that living in a neighbourhood which encourages an
unfamiliar lifestyle, culture and language is a risk factor for
the development of mental disorder. Of course categorizing
people as black or white and assuming that all blacks and all
whites identify with their own ethnic culture is a gross
simplification. Furthermore, as cultural minorities become

more established in 'good' areas, the assumed monocultural white ethos of these communities will presumably diminish. However, throughout the world, and especially the world's major cities, we continue to find areas which are synonymous with one cultural group or another. For example, most major cities of the 'Western' world now have Chinese, French, Indian and Italian districts. There now appears to be good evidence that people who live in communities which are characterized by a large number of members of their own cultural group experience a feeling of 'fitting in'.

What prevents the negative effects of cultural isolation appears not to be the absolute number of other members of your cultural group, but their number *relative* to other groups. Interestingly the high rates of admission to psychiatric facilities found in British Afro-Caribbeans is not so characteristic of Indian and Pakistani communities in Britain. Halpern (1993) reviews research which suggests that this can be accounted for by the differing tendencies of these groups to 'cluster'. Apparently, a geographical analysis of immigrant settlement in Britain reveals that Asians have tended to cluster more than West Indians. Such segregation may help to protect the members of Asian communities from direct prejudice and provide them with social support which operates through culturally familiar customs.

As described in the introductory chapter of this book, social psychology emphasizes how an individual personally gains from being an accepted member of a group. Individuals may define themselves with reference to their cultural group, feel empowered by being a member of that group and evaluate themselves in relation to other people within the group. If members of a cultural group live far apart geographically (low density) they may become less able to identify with membership of it. Other factors, interests or demands will impinge on their experience of life. Their sense of a cultural community will dissipate and they may become less able to deal with their problems. In this way, both geographically and psychologically, their loss of a sense of community may predispose them to mental disorder. Halpern's 'cultural density' theory should therefore be central to the clinician's endeavours to create health through the management of community resources. As Halpern concludes: 'to dwell amongst members of the same perceived group offers some kind of perceived psychological advantage' (1993, p. 605).

## Personality disorder

Cultures are the products of different ways of 'being' in the world. Cultures describe the ways in which groups of people experience, think, feel and behave. Within cultures, at the level of the individual, there are also different ways of experiencing, thinking, feeling and behaving. These individual differences form the basis of individuals' personalities. It is the variation of personalities within a culture which makes stereotyping an erroneous method of dealing with people. Yet it is undeniable that cultures differ in what characterizes their customary behaviour. A widely accepted notion within personality theory is that childhood experiences influence subsequent personality development. It is therefore reasonable to assume that cultural variations in family life and gender role, for instance, will have an influence on the sort of personalities which develop, in order to adapt to the customary requirements of their culture. In short, different cultures place different expectations on individuals and make different allowances for individuals.

Culture has a strong influence on the construction of a self-concept, for by comparing ourselves with other people we are able to 'describe' ourselves: 'I am sensitive like Mary', 'I have a bad temper, much worse than Jimmy's', 'I am not as attractive as Liz'. Culture does not only help us place ourselves in relation to other people and/or ideas, it also delineates what is good or bad, mad or sad. Culture conveys certain expectations of normative behaviour: it defines normality and abnormality. It is in this sense that cultural differences are especially salient for personality disorders. In a recent review Alarcon and Foulks (1995) have suggested that a personality disorder (PD) 'reflects difficulties in how an individual behaves and is perceived to behave by others in the social field, and this, of necessity, brings into play cultural values related to what is expected, valued, and devalued in a person' (p.6). If PDs concern failing to adapt to, or function in, certain situations then they are clearly related to culture. Deviance from the culturally expected, or 'normal', personality may define disorder and dysfunction. Awareness of this has led to a concern for 'culturally contextualizing' behaviour: understanding it in its cultural context.

The prevailing understanding of PDs is based on a 'Western' understanding of behaviour which promotes active, autonomous and self-reliant behaviour. The 'Western' conception of the 'ideal person' probably also incorporates the Protestant work ethic, the accumulation of wealth, scientific rationality and so on. Such values also contribute to definitions of people who are on the margins of a culture, people who have PDs. Alarcon and Foulks describe how many of the traits included in contemporary psychiatric diagnoses (in particular DSM-IV) may be considered quite appropriate in other cultures. In Table 4.4 I have extracted from their review to give some idea of culturally appropriate behaviours that could be clinically misleading and therefore misclassified as indicating a personality disorder. When reading Table 4.4 it is worth bearing in mind that DSM-IV is a product of the *American* Psychiatric Association. It therefore reflects American (often white, middle class, Anglo American) views of behaviours which are not common or desired in that (sub)culture.

A few of the examples in Table 4.4 deserve further comment. The possibly traumatic experience of migration and acculturation may lead to behaviours which others interpret as signs of paranoid, schizoid, antisocial or avoidant personality disorder. This is saying nothing more than some immigrants do not

**Table 4.4:** Culturally normative behaviours which may be clinically misleading and misclassified as Personality Disorder (PD) according to DSM–IV criteria

| Examples of behaviour | Cultures/contexts in which it is normative | DSM–IV diagnosis |
|---|---|---|
| Secretive, mistrustful, self-protective | Arabs, Mediterraneans, Eastern Europeans, Immigrants | Paranoid PD |
| Social isolation, indifference to society, communicative deficits | Rural-to-urban and international migration | Schizoid PD |
| Peculiar ideation, appearance, 'speaking in tongues' | Evangelical religions, Native Americans, Hispanics | Schizotypal PD |
| Displays of tension, conflict, antagonism, dysphoria | Welfare activists in deprived communities, immigrants from 'oppressed countries' | Antisocial PD |
| Suicidal-like behaviour such as wrist-slashing | Native and Asian Americans and Arabs | Border-line PD |
| Emotionality, seductiveness, self-centredness, dramatic, hypersociability, somatization | Mediterraneans and people of Latin descent | Histrionic PD |
| Flamboyance, self-importance, self-aggrandizement | Ethnic groups of Latin descent | Narcissistic PD |
| Distrust of officialdom, poor self-efficacy, demoralization, oversensitivity, suppression of affect | Oppressed or minority groups especially Asian, Filipino and Hispanic immigrants | Avoidant PD |
| Passivity, deferential, faith in authority figures and elders | Traditional Asians and Arctic groups | Dependent PD |
| Strong work ethic, intolerance, inflexibility, judgemental | Scholars, scientists, priests, Japanese | Obsessive-Compulsive PD |

Based on Alarcon and Foulks' (1995), literature review.

know, or have not adopted, the culturally acceptable ways of behaving as implied by DSM-IV. Ethnic groups who are 'settled' into mainstream society and yet retain aspects of their original cultural identity, also run the risk of being misunderstood. Wrist slashing among Native and Asian Americans would be a good example of this. In some Native American cultures this behaviour is a method of achieving bonding. The closest approximation to this behaviour in mainstream American culture occurs as suicidal behaviour often associated with aggression and is therefore associated with borderline PD.

As a final comment on Table 4.4 it is important to emphasize how some apparently prosocial (positive) behaviours can also fall foul of psychiatric classification. For instance, the behaviour of an Italian lady who is extremely sociable, dramatic and seductive (prosocial?) could be interpreted as symptomatic of histrionic PD. For example, I know a number of women who would feel that their holidays were completely wasted if Italian men did not behave in this manner! Personality disorders are about misbehaving in certain contexts; they are about not knowing of, or abiding by, certain social norms. This difficulty can reflect great mental distress and require appropriate intervention to alleviate an individual's suffering. It is therefore all the more important not to confuse behaviours characteristic of some cultures or contexts with the diagnosis of 'Western' suffering. To do so dilutes the validity of true personality disorder and affronts the lifestyles of people from 'non-Western' cultures.

## TRANSITION MENTAL HEALTH

I have tried to emphasize the importance of keeping the individual characteristics of people in the foreground while acknowledging the broader social and cultural factors as the context in which individuals operate. It is important not to stereotype an individual by over-identifying him or her with a particular cultural persona. In the same way we must avoid making easy assumptions about people who can be easily grouped together. For instance, 'refugees', 'the elderly', 'the handicapped' and so on. Yet it is also important to acknowledge that, to the extent that people share common problems or situations, then an awareness of these can be helpful in understanding their health needs. The aim here is only to touch on certain issues relevant to clinical practice so as to create awareness and hopefully motivate further reading, reflection and research, so that clinicians can explore those issues in their own practice.

## TRANSITIONS

Transition refers to change. The changes which accompany resettlement can be many and varied. An emigrant is someone who leaves a place in which he or she has been settled; an immigrant is someone who arrives to resettle in a new place. Thus the same individual will be both an emigrant and an immigrant depending on whether he or she is coming or going. This process of change is referred to as migration.

## Migration

Contemporary migrations are on a scale and of a diversity previously unknown. The World Bank has estimated that the number of international migrants now exceed 100 million and migration is now recognized as a global challenge. The United Nations Populations Fund (UNFPA) made migration the main issue of its 1993 World Population Report. The urbanization of many cultures has come about as a result of economic and industrial pressure to centralize resources. With the mechanization of agricultural production and in many countries, the decreasing proportion of Gross National Product (GNP) that is constituted by agriculture, there has been a decline in rural populations. Thus within many countries there has been, and continues to be, a major migration from rural to urban areas. International migration is also now occurring on an unprecedented scale, with the proportion of people living outside their country of birth now approaching 2 per cent. This migration, of course, occurs for many different reasons but is, in the majority of cases, in one direction.

From 1980 to 1992, 15 million people migrated to Europe, mainly for permanent settlement. Now the dominant movement is from 'Eastern' Europe and the former Soviet Union into 'Western' Europe and North America. Patterns of migration in Central America and the Caribbean have been dominated by movement to the United States, Brazil and Venezuela. Since the 1960s the oil-producing countries have attracted migrant labour from 'Middle Eastern' and Asian countries. However, the emergence of strong economies in east and southeast Asia (for instance, Japan, Singapore and the Republic of Korea) has also recently drawn migrants from poorer countries in the region (such as Bangladesh, the Philippines and Indonesia), while other Asians have migrated to the 'melting pots' of Europe, North America and Australia. In southern Africa there has been considerable migration to South Africa, while in northern Africa there has been much migration to Europe.

Patterns of migration reflect changes in the economic, social and cultural relationships between different peoples. However, the combinations of poverty, rapid population growth and environmental damage (for example, soil erosion) often create instability, resulting in the outpouring of people. While once immigrants were viewed as extra workers for a thriving economy, now they may be viewed as a threat to the security and well-being of local workers and to the recipient society at large. Also, previously many migrants were men, now women and children form a substantial proportion of migrants. This has heightened the role of gender in migration. While both men and women migrants often experience 'downward occupational mobility' (working at a lower level than they were trained for in their own country) this effect appears to be much stronger for women. Women have also had to confront the dilemmas which radically different cultural expectations of their role, in their 'home' country and their host country, may present. At another extreme, people from industrially rich countries may emigrate to poorer countries in search of a better life. In Hawaii, the 'coconuts and bananas syndrome', refers to the expectation among some migrants that life there will be easier, more simple, with luscious foods dropping into their hands from nearby trees!

Whatever the reasons for migration, some of the experience of transition will be shared by different groups. Table 4.5 summarizes some of these common themes as described by Westermeyer (1989) in his book on refugees and migrants. Some of these are more obvious than others. For instance, 'delayed cultural conflict' refers to those people who may have successfully adjusted to life in a different culture on a day-to-day basis, but who again experience conflict at irregular events such as funerals, weddings, childbirth and so on. Such events may embody quite different symbolic meanings in different cultures. 'Life cycle changes' may result in intergenerational conflicts. For instance, immigrant children, due to their more rapid language acquisition and possibly easier entry into a new culture, may serve as translators and socializers for their parents and grandparents. Such role-reversal may be stressful for all those concerned. 'Loyalties' to past commitments and to the demands of the present may be in conflict. One rather abstract example of this is if, in order to become a national of a new country, one has to renounce citizenship of one's country of origin. 'Returning home' may be an unexpectedly stressful experience for some emigrants. Often they themselves have changed and others may find it difficult to slot them back into what was once their familiar social network.

## Causes and precipitants of mental disorder in migrants

It is not surprising then to find that the experience of migration, with the necessary adaption to a new life context, can be

**Table 4.5:** Changes associated with migration

| | |
|---|---|
| Attitudes/values/beliefs/mores | Laws/regulations/legal status |
| Recreational activities | Loyalties |
| Circadian rhythms | Religious practices |
| Communication | Returning home |
| Delayed culture conflicts | Social network loss |
| Developmental/life cycle changes | Social roles |
| Ecological changes | Vocational changes |

After Westermeyer (1989).

stressful. However, research has shown that various factors influence the degree to which this stress may result in significant psychological disorder. Table 4.6 summarizes the causes and precipitants of such disorder, once again, as described by Westermeyer. While some of the factors in Table 4.6 will affect most forms of migration (e.g. exchange college students, refugees, immigrants from the 'Third' world) others will be particular to some types, and yet others can be found exerting deleterious affects in non-migrants too. Table 4.6 omits other factors which might be expected to cause mental distress or disorder in anybody (for example, certain genetic, biomedical, environmental or familial factors) and focuses on those which are particularly relevant to the experience of migration. Such migrations could include refugees, guest workers (*gastarbeiter*), permanent emigrants, students studying abroad, temporary expatriate workers and so on. The unifying theme among them all is one of transition between cultures. Some of the factors reviewed below will be more relevant to some groups than to others.

### Premigration factors

Self-selection, or the 'Drift Hypothesis', refers to the notion that migration may be particularly attractive to people who are predisposed to mental disorder. Following on from this is the idea of biased migration where a country actually facilitates the migration of its least desirable citizens (e.g. paupers,

**Table 4.6:** Causes and precipitants of mental disorder in migrants

| *Premigration factors* | *Family factors* |
|---|---|
| Self-selection (drift hypothesis) | Absence of family/partial |
| Biased migration | family |
| Forced migration | Family expectations |
| National policy | Marital conflict |
| Traumatic events | Intergenerational conflict |
| Lack of preparation | |
| | *Psychological factors* |
| *Cultural factors* | Loss and grief |
| Culture shock | Guilt and shame |
| Future shock | Status inconsistency |
| Demodernization shock | Maladaptive traditionality |
| Language and communication | Life change events |
| Acculturation stresses | Attitudes |
| Minority status | Expectations |
| | Homesickness |
| *Social factors* | |
| Loss of social network | *Biological factors* |
| Social isolation | Acute travel effects |
| Role strain | Organic brain damage |
| Marginality | Chronic illness |
| Unemployment | Growing old |
| Prejudice/bigotry | |
| Iatrogenic morbidity | |

After Westermeyer (1989).

criminals, the chronically mentally disordered). Forced migration may occur to escape death, imprisonment or poverty, for instance, and it seems to be the case that the more involuntary a migration is, then the more likely it is to act as a precipitating factor in mental disorder. Migration as a national policy does not necessarily imply that it need be official government policy. For instance, many Irish university graduates migrate each year because of difficulties in finding employment within Ireland, yet there are no attempts to cut back on the number of graduates the state produces. Thus migration may be seen as a default policy. Perhaps the other end of the spectrum is migration which results from traumatic events. This is commonly associated with the migration of political prisoners or refugees and may present in various stress-related reactions, including post-traumatic stress disorder (PTSD). The final premigration factor described by Westermeyer is lack of preparation. Desirable preparation may include language training, prior experience of separation from those left behind, a plan for acculturation, and so on.

### Cultural factors

A number of cultural factors may explicitly cause or precipitate mental disorder. 'Culture shock' has already been described. 'Future shock' refers to the rapid technological advancement and social changes which many societies are experiencing. These changes may be unsettling, disorientating and unintegrated, especially when encountered through migration as opposed to 'accelerated modernization', which may also present challenges to social relationships and personal well-being. Demodernization stress can occur when people fail to adapt to their new environment. For example, immigrants from tropical areas who fail to adapt their dress to colder northern climates may experience frostbite, while those from northern climates who migrate to tropical areas may risk dehydration and heat stroke by failing to dress appropriately. Similarly, moving from humid to arid areas (or vice versa), or from low to high latitudes, each has various maladies associated with them. Perhaps more expectedly the term 'demodernization stress' also describes the difficulties encountered when an individual moves from what he or she considers to be a 'more modern' (usually technologically sophisticated) to 'less modern' environment. We have already reviewed the importance of language/ communication including verbal and non-verbal communications. 'Acculturation stresses' refers to the conflicts in the long-term adjustment to a new system of living and has also been described in Chapter 2. Finally, minority status is often a new experience for many migrants who originate from places where 'their type' is in the majority. This new status

may single the individual out as different and through prejudice of the majority, or fear within the minority, produce
many concomitant stresses.

### *Social factors*

A related but distinguishable category of causes and
precipitating factors for mental disorder is social factors.
Migration usually involves the loss of an individual's social
network and this will obviously influence the amount of
social support available to a person which might enable
them to cope more effectively with a stressful situation.
Social isolation may therefore not only be stressful in itself
but may also act as a vulnerability factor. Such isolation may
be heightened unless immigrants move into areas where
'their type' are accepted. Role strain may occur where people
are attempting to fulfil roles (e.g. work roles) which their
background, experience, or more generally their culture, has
not prepared them for. For instance, women from cultures
which have traditionally put them in the role of homemaker,
may struggle to adapt to the role of factory worker. Also,
similar social roles in their country of origin and in their new
country may involve quite different skills. The process of
transition may also result in a person no longer feeling themselves to be part of a group. This 'marginality' may become a
dual-marginality if an immigrant neither identifies with their
own ethnic group or with that of the place they have moved
into.

Unemployment may be a major stressor because it can
encompass many other negative factors such as poverty, lack
of an occupational role, lack of social network, lack of
opportunities to maintain or enhance self-esteem and so on.
Prejudice and bigotry will inevitably lead to increased
psychological burden on immigrants. It is likely to be at its
worst in situations of high local unemployment,
communities with little cultural diversity, communities with
a history of domination by one cultural group and where

unwritten rules about access of certain cultural groups to particular areas, residences, jobs, etc., apply. The last example listed by Westermeyer under the social category is 'iatrogenic morbidity'. Iatrogenic refers to the induction of further (or a different type of) distress or illness in a person as a result of a clinician's attempts to treat that person. Westermeyer argues that treating people from different cultures may result in failures to communicate different understandings surrounding their problems (that is, diagnosis, treatment, expectations of each other, etc.), and when coupled with factors such as poor social support, may result in worsening or additional problems for the person. The importance of such communication is discussed further in Chapter 6.

### Family factors

Various factors relating more directly to the family may also cause or precipitate mental disorder. Sharing the same past, the same migration and the same new environment can strengthen family relationships, while solo migration, or migration of only some members of the family, reduces this potentially positive effect and may psychologically distance family members from each other. However, family expectations of, for instance, a son excelling academically at a university abroad, or of a daughter sending money back home, may place significant additional demands on the migrant. As well as this, the (different) experiences of migratory transitions can place strain on close relationships, as can being separated from a partner for months or years. Different acculturation experiences may also relate to age, with younger people finding it easier to adapt to the different lifestyle of a new culture, than do older people. Also many immigrants may leave behind a society where being older is associated with greater wisdom and being shown more respect, and enter into a society where the elderly are seen as 'spent'. Naturally such a change in status can be very distressing and fuel intergenerational conflicts.

### Psychological factors

For those migrating permanently or for prolonged periods a sense of loss and grieving after what has been left behind, including a particular self-identity, is a common reaction. Homesickness, obsessively longing after their 'home', may be an aspect of this. Self-perception may also be an important issue for those with experiences of combat or civil unrest, where they may feel guilt or shame concerning their own behaviour. Status inconsistency (already discussed), and the difficulties of integrating a meaningful self-concept because of this, may produce significant stress for an individual. Sometimes people will continue to identify with the place they have migrated from. This reluctance to redefine oneself, 'maladaptive traditionality', may prohibit opportunities to enjoy life in a new culture. Psychological research has highlighted how an accumulation of negative life change events (for instance, divorce, unemployment or the loss of a loved one), or, indeed, positive life change events (such as marriage, childbirth or promotion in work), can be detrimental to health, especially for those already low in self-esteem.

Clearly the experience of migration not only includes a massive array of life changes but also, as has been mentioned, often can reduce personal resources to deal with such changes. Westermeyer also notes some potentially troublesome attitudes and expectations among some migrants. In the case of victims of premigration horrors he suggests that they sometimes behave as though they are owed or entitled to something as a result of their unjust persecutions. Also they may project their hostility towards their persecutors as rage against those who are now trying to alleviate their suffering. Such individuals may also have unrealistically idealized expectations of what their new country can offer them.

### Biological factors

The acute travel effects of the migratory experience are often overlooked. Travel across time zones may produce fatigue, hypoxia in jet flights, dehydration and a plethora of other experiences which can exacerbate existing problems and stressors. In certain types of migration, where people have experienced extreme deprivation or dangerous environments—malnutrition, famine, hyperthermia, hypothermia, untreated infections, war wounds and so on—these may have led to organic brain damage. Similarly, unborn infants exposed to such problems *in utero*, as well as infants and children, may also develop organic brain damage. Add to this the presence of certain dangerous diseases which may be endemic to areas that emigrants leave (for instance, malaria or measles) and it can be seen that organic disorders may also be an important factor in precipitating or causing mental disorder. Chronic physical illnesses may also be more difficult to cope with and therefore worsen in unfamiliar environments, especially where these are associated with a reduction in social support. The relevance of old age to migration has already been mentioned in a number of contexts; it is, however, noteworthy that several North American research studies have found that elderly migrants have a higher rate of psychiatric hospitalization than elderly native-born 'Americans'. The reasons for this are not clear but may well relate more to the psychosocial factors (described above) than to strictly biological ones (Westermeyer, 1989).

Other factors could surely be added to Westermeyer's list and some people would argue about the relative strength and prevalence of the factors presented here. However, there should be no attempt to neglect the diversity which exists within any group of refugees, students, sojourners, gastarbeiter, tourists or whoever by developing a caricature of them. I see Westermeyer's list of factors as a useful checklist of issues which may be influencing how well people are adapting to their migration experience and how this may interact with their health, mental and physical. As we have focused on mental aspects of migration let us briefly consider how these may interact with physical well-being.

### Cancer and the stress of immigration

From the end of 1989 to June 1992, 380,152 Jews from the former Soviet Union emigrated to Israel, increasing that country's population by almost 10 per cent. Adverse conditions in the Soviet Union, such as political instability, economic hardship, national conflicts and fear of increasing anti-Semitism motivated these migrants, many of whom knew very little about Israel. In Israel they confronted severe housing shortages and high levels of unemployment, along with the radically different culture of Israel. During this time, Baider and colleagues (1996), from Hadassah University in Jerusalem, studied the adjustment and psychological distress of 116 of these immigrants who had cancer and compared them to 288 healthy immigrants who had also come from the former Soviet Union.

They found that all immigrants, whether physically healthy or not, reported significant adjustment problems. Sixty per cent of the physically healthy group reported that their employment, economic and social conditions were *worse* in Israel than in Russia. Among the cancer patients this was even stronger with almost 80 per cent judging their social situation in Israel to be worse than it was in Russia. Both groups scored highly in terms of mental distress, with the mean score in both the male and female cancer patients exceeding the cut-off (on the Brief Symptom Inventory) for mental disorder 'caseness'. The average age of cancer patients was significantly higher than that of the physically healthy control group and this factor might also have contributed to their distress in that they may have been less adaptable. Also, the majority (almost 90 per cent) of the cancer patients had been diagnosed since arriving in Israel. Putting all of these factors together—recent serious diagnosis, being older, recently arriving in a new country, being out of work, economically worse off and possibly having less social support—we can appreciate that the health of these migrants was influenced by many more factors than having to adapt to a different culture. So it is with any cultural group entering into a different culture. They do not only bring their culture with them but also a plethora of demographic and psychosocial factors which may place them at risk and make their recovery more problematic.

The study by Baider and colleagues further illustrates the complexity of the health of immigrants in its findings regarding social support. It is well recognized that social support, especially support from the spouse, can be of great benefit to people attempting to cope with cancer. For the male patients in Braider et al.'s study, and for both the healthy male and female immigrants, the perception of strong family support was associated with less distress. Not so for the female cancer patients, where there was no significant relationship between the level of perceived family support and psychological well-being. It may therefore be very important to note such a gender difference (also reported in other studies of adjustment to chronic disease) in designing interventions for such immigrants groups. While illustrating the complexity of individual differences within an immigrant group, Baider et al.'s general conclusion seems justified: '. . . cancer patients who have to cope with an additional stress (immigration in this study) should be regarded as highly vulnerable patients who, as a consequence, develop extreme psychological distress' (1996, p. 1082).

## Refugees

Physical symptoms and distress may also be an aspect of the migration experience, even when these are not associated with premigration illness. We now review some interesting German research on this topic. With one inhabitant in every 50 being a refugee, Germany has one of the highest proportions of refugees to nationals in the world. In 1992 its 1.6 million refugees included recognized asylum seekers (6 per cent) and their dependants (8 per cent), quota refugees (5 per cent) accepted on account of international humanitarian

actions, asylum seekers (i.e. applicants, 37 per cent) and *de-
facto* refugees (44 per cent), that is, people without right of
asylum but who were not expelled for humanitarian or political reasons. Again this sort of breakdown illustrates that refugees are not a homogeneous group and that entitlement to
'refugee status', which may carry with it benefits of access to
health and welfare services, does not accrue to every individual seeking refuge in a foreign country.

Schwarzer and colleagues (1994), from the Free University of
Berlin, investigated the effects of prolonged unemployment
and lack of social support among 235 East German refugees.
In fact, while the majority of their sample were indeed refugees (62 per cent of them having come to West Berlin before
the opening of the Berlin Wall on 9 November 1989), the
remaining 38 per cent were technically legal migrants as they
arrived after this date. These two groups were, however,
treated together since there were no significant psychological
differences between the two groups (in statistical terms).

The outcome variable for the study was a 24-item self-report
measure of physical symptoms including heart complaints,
pains in the limbs, stomach complaints and exhaustion. Each
item was scored on a 5-point Likert-type scale. Measures of
physical symptoms, social support and employment status
were taken at three different times over the two years following their transition to West Berlin. Those who were always
jobless over the two-year period reported significantly more
physical symptoms than those who were employed. Also,
those who received less social support (determined by a me-
dian split) reported significantly more physical symptoms
that those who received more social support. However, the
really interesting question was: How would these factors interact? Figure 4.1, which graphs these results, illustrates a
significant interaction between employment status and social
support. Those who experienced both unemployment and
relatively low levels of social support reported the highest
levels of physical symptoms at each of the three points of

**Illness**

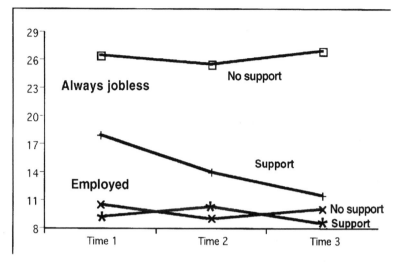

**Figure 4.1:** Employment, social support and physical symptoms among East German 'refugees' (reproduced from Schwarzer *et al.*, 1994, with permission)

measurement. Those who remained jobless from Time 1 to Time 3, but who received high levels of social support, showed a dramatic decline in reported physical symptoms over time. This effect appears to reflect the 'buffer' effect of social support; that is, receiving a high level of social support buffers, or reduces, the detrimental effects which stress can have on health.

It is clearly desirable for refugees, migrants or anyone else entering a new society to have the opportunity for employment. Employment not only gives economic benefits but it also provides psychological benefits through giving a sense of purpose and social benefits as a result of the social role(s) which go along with a job. In addition to this, it also acts as a gateway to social support from colleagues. The unfortunate reality is that many immigrants find it very difficult to get a job in their new country, at least initially. Studies such as that by Schwarzer and colleagues illustrate how unemployed immigrants living in communities which afford them little social support are likely to experience more symptoms of physical illness. It is also quite possible that this increased level of illness will ultimately place greater demands on health services than would be the case if more social support was available.

On the basis of this line of argument it is therefore very important for health professionals to actively advocate the settlement of immigrants in environments which will afford them the maximum social support and therefore the maximum buffer against the development of certain physical symptoms. The health of people travelling across cultures is not simply determined by what they have left behind them or by what they bring with them, but also by how they are received. Their reception into communities capable of providing meaningful social support may be the greatest help that we as clinicians can give them. It should not be assumed that such a community will necessarily be a clone of their culture of origin, for other research suggests that too strong an identification with the culture of origin may make the acculturative experience more stressful (see Dona & Berry, 1994). Nonetheless, the social context into which immigrants are expected to commune must be one which knows how to welcome, embrace and support its new members in ways which recognize their customs. As a final perspective on refugeehood, the case study below describes the situation of a refugee family after leaving their home country. It conveys something of the circumstances refugees may have left behind them before becoming permanent residents in another country.

---

### Case Study: Running from Fear

*The following referral letter is based on my own case material. The letter was addressed to a Senior Protection Officer, resident at a*

*United Nations High Commissioner for Refugees (UNHCR) office, and recommends that UNHCR evacuates a family to elsewhere. [All names and locations have been changed.]*

*Mr S. Naik,*
*Senior Protection Officer,*
*UNHCR,*
*. . .*

*Dear Mr Naik,*

*At the request of an official of the Baptist Church in Bowali, I interviewed Mr and Mrs Mzimba on 10 June in order to assess their mental state.*

*Mr and Mrs Mzimba and their five children have been refugees for some time. They experienced the trauma of imperative forced flight from their country of origin and several subsequent relocations. They have had difficulties integrating with local and refugee communities because of a continuing fear for their safety. They are concerned that certain factions from their country of origin are attempting to trace them with the purpose of killing them. The fact that close friends of theirs who were forced to leave the same country recently died under suspicious circumstances, appears to give some credence to their fears. The Mzimbas, who might otherwise be expected to make a meaningful contribution to society, find themselves in a state of insecurity, bewilderment, disorientation and alienation.*

*In the case of Mrs Mzimba this has recently driven her to attempt suicide. She has also expressed the idea of 'saving her children from the world'. At interview she presented with depressed affect and reported feelings of pessimism and helplessness. In addition I understand that she has been confused and disorientated in the past few weeks. Mr Mzimba has been a constant source of support and strength to his wife throughout their exile. However, I feel that the pressures of this commitment are now beginning to affect his own judgement and that he is floundering; reporting both anxious and depressive experiences. In my estimation there is a real and frightening potential for self-destruction within the family. They continue to struggle with their perceived insecurity and an environment which offers little support and no realistic prospects of employment. There is very little professional support available to the Mzimbas in the town of Bowali, the Mzimbas do not speak the local language and there are significant cultural differences between this country and their country of origin.*

*I strongly recommend that the Mzimba family be evacuated to a secure environment which can provide the level of professional support they require. Being fluent in English they have expressed a wish to be sent to an English-speaking country which has some experience in receiving refugees. I would like to end on a positive note by saying that Mr and Mrs Mzimba are clearly intelligent people with the ability to make a genuine contribution to a host society, rather than simply being 'accommodated' by one. I believe that in time a recipient country would benefit from accepting them . . .*

*Your sincerely,*

Unfortunately in the case of the Mzimbas, although they were evacuated to an English-speaking country, they had great difficulties in obtaining any sort of employment. They found it impossible to gain employment at an equivalent level of professionalism that they were employed at in their own country. Such factors may have a profound effect on their health, for, as we have seen, social support and employment may influence the psychological stress associated with pre-existing problems.

## CONCLUSION

In this chapter we considered the complexities of charting depression across different cultures. Considering a particular disorder from different cultural perspectives can sharpen one's understanding and it can also question one's assumptions. It is when we see our own society as one of many cultures that we can then operate most effectively as multicultural practitioners. This perspective is vital if we are to avoid making serious errors in the hazardous diagnosis of conditions such as personality disorder, where being exposed to the 'right' kind of socialization may be very important. The social context of mental health is nowhere more clearly represented than in the plight of many minority immigrant groups who live in social, political and economic disadvantage. Yet these factors, and culture, do not partition our experience of the world into neat 'mental' and 'physical' boxes; instead they are each part of the same experience. In Chapter 5 we consider the physical aspect of culture and our experience of health.

## GUIDELINES FOR PROFESSIONAL PRACTICE

1. Research on cross-cultural mental health is very diverse and includes comparative, cultural minority and transitional approaches. While there is overlap between these areas of research they are undertaken with different questions in mind and in different contexts and settings. It may not, therefore, be legitimate to generalize results derived from one of these approaches to problems encountered in another approach.
2. Clinicians should avoid the temptation to assimilate an unfamiliar form of suffering into a familiar diagnostic system. An example of this may be seen in attempts to 'fit' a range of somatic symptoms (which occur in many and diverse cultures) into the diagnostic category of depression.
3. Clinicians should attempt to understand the meaning of a person's problem within that person's terms of reference. Such 'terms of reference' are likely to reflect not only cultural norms but also social, economic and political factors.

4. Cultural identity is a community resource which is relevant to health care. The individuals within a community may be healthier if their culture is in the majority or is at least a sizeable minority. Clinicians should inform people of the possible negative health consequences of moving from communities where their cultural group is in the majority to communities where their cultural group is in the minority. Higher rates of psychological disturbance appear to be associated with group minority status.

5. The use of 'Western-based' diagnostic systems may misclassify certain cultural behaviours as disorders. An example of this is the category of personality disorder which describes socially inappropriate ways of behaving within most 'Western' cultures. Clinicians should seek to understand the intended function of unusual behaviours and explore the extent to which the observed behaviour might be functional within their client's culture.

6. The experience of transition may constitute a serious stressor in itself and/or may aggravate existing mental and physical health problems. A number of factors detailed in Table 4.6 may be related to the onset of migration-related disorder.

7. Migration not only involves a change of cultural settings but also economic, political and social factors which may all impact on health. Clinicians should broaden their own frame of reference to include the many factors which impinge upon an individual's health. While individual clinicians may not be able to influence many of the broader issues directly, the clinician's acknowledgement of them can legitimize the distress experienced by their clients.

# 5

# CULTURE AND PHYSICAL HEALTH

This chapter reviews the influence which cultural differences may have on physical health. It is once again worth emphasizing that cultural differences do not occur in isolation. They can be associated with socioeconomic, environmental, dietary, behavioural and genetic variations. It is therefore often a matter of relating physical health to cultural variation through one of these routes. For instance, the relatively high incidence of sickle-cell anaemia among west African men can be attributed to genetic factors. Different 'dietary cultures' may also account for the high incidence of rickets in some immigrant groups. The effects of dietary variations are also evident in the well-known difficulties which Chinese people have in metabolizing milk-based products, or which Europeans have in dealing with a genuine Vindaloo curry! However, before reviewing this literature I would like to argue for culture having a much broader impact on physical health than suggested above. There are two aspects to this argument. The first is that psychosocial processes influence physical health. The second is that some cultural differences also relate to health (perhaps through the psychosocial processes which have been shown to be important). Following our review of these issues we consider the extent to which cultural groups may differ in their health problems, whether cultures understand the physical body in different ways and how different cultures react to various diseases.

## PSYCHOSOCIAL PROCESSES AND PHYSICAL HEALTH

Steptoe (1991) has described three ways in which psychological and social factors can be linked to physical disease states. The first of these, **psychophysiological hyperactivity,** refers to the effects which continuous stress can produce on the body. Many people react similarly to severe momentary stress with, for instance, palpitations, sweating, breathlessness and perhaps trembling. However, if an individual is continuously in a stressful environment this level of physiological responding cannot be sustained. Physiological arousal therefore declines and there may be few visible signs of stress. Nonetheless, the body is in quite a different physiological state than when it is relaxed. After prolonged stress and the attempts of the body's systems to adapt to their increased physiological demands, the body becomes depleted of its ability to fight off infection and to supply its various organs with sufficient resources. Physiological damage may occur in any of the body's systems or organs. Individuals differ in the physiological problems which they develop in response to prolonged stress. It is almost as though we have a physiological 'Achilles' heel'; a relative weakness in our physiological make up which is therefore relatively more vulnerable to the effects of prolonged stress.

Psychosocial processes may also be linked to disease through their influence on **disease stability and progression.** In this case we are not talking of psychosocial causes of disease but instead of how psychosocial processes may influence existing disease, whatever its cause. For instance, people may suffer from asthma, but exactly when they have an asthma attack or how severe the attack is can be influenced by psychosocial factors such as the degree of stress in their immediate environment.

A third way in which psychosocial factors are linked with disease is through their influence on **host vulnerability.** In

this case the physiological effects of stress have no direct influence on disease. However, as described above, the prolonged effects of stress deplete the resources of the body. One
aspect of this is that the body's immune system is suppressed
so that its ability to fight off invasive pathogens is diminished.
The body becomes more susceptible to infections. For instance, it has been found that people are more likely to
develop a common cold when they are under stress than
when they are not. Although there are 'colds' out there all the
time, usually we are able to fight them off. Thus stress doesn't
give you the 'cold', but should you encounter the cold virus, it
makes you more vulnerable to it.

There is now a convincing literature to support the existence
of the above pathways between psychosocial processes and
physical disease. In addition, Steptoe and Wardle (1994) have
recently brought together a collection of scientific papers,
published over the last 30 years, which relate to the influence
that psychosocial processes have on physical health and illness. In order to illustrate these influences in summary, Table
5.1 depicts some of the relationships revealed in these papers.
As can be seen, a great range of different factors are associated with physical welfare and ailments. Some of these relationships are of a rather general nature, for instance, higher
rates of mortality (from whatever cause) being associated
with unemployment, small social networks and the suppression of anger. Likewise, physical illness (from whatever
cause) is associated with whether people explain events in an
optimistic or pessimistic manner, the amount of control they
have over their environment and their degree of 'hardiness'.
'Hardiness' refers to the extent to which people will respond
to a stressful situation by (1) believing that they can exert
personal control over it, (2) demonstrating a commitment to
solving the problem and (3) seeing the situation as a challenge
rather than as a threat (Kobasa *et al.*, 1985).

More specific relationships have also been identified. These
include the conjunction of undesirable events and frustration

**Table 5.1:** Psychological factors with demonstrated relationships to
physical health

| Psychosocial factor | Physical state | Source* |
| --- | --- | --- |
| Unemployment | Mortality (by any cause), cardiovascular disease, cancer | Moser *et al.* (1984) |
| Job strain and work-related social support | Cardiovascular disease | Johnson *et al.* (1988) |
| Small social networks | Mortality (by any cause) | Berkman and Syme (1979) |
| Goal frustration and negative life events | Gastrointestinal disorders | Craig and Brown (1984) |
| Poor coping resources and negative life events | Pregnancy complications | Nuckolls *et al.* (1972) |
| Psychological stress | Myocardial ischemia | Rozanski *et al.* (1991) |
| Psychological stress | Common cold | Cohen *et al.* (1991) |
| Type-A behaviour | Coronary heart disease | Rosenman *et al.* (1975) |
| Bereavement | Lymphocyte function | Bartrop *et al.* (1977) |
| Anger suppression | Mortality (by any cause) | Julius *et al.* (1986) |
| Pessimistic explanatory style | Physical illness (any type) | Peterson *et al.* (1988) |
| Hardiness | Physical illness (any type) | Ouellette *et al.* (1985) |

* All of these research papers can be found in Steptoe and Wardle (1994).

over not being able to achieve personal goals, predicting gastrointestinal disorders such as an ulcer. Poor coping resources, also in conjunction with undesirable events, have been found to predict complications in pregnancy; bereavement is associated with a reduction in lymphocyte function, and high levels of mental stress are linked to poor cardiovascular functioning. While some relationships, such as that between 'type A behaviour' and coronary heart disease, may remain controversial, others are now much clearer. However, taken together, as a body of evidence, this research weighs strongly in favour of accepting the first point outlined in the introduction, that psychosocial processes do indeed have an influence on physical health.

## CULTURAL DIFFERENCES AND PHYSICAL HEALTH

We have already reviewed in Chapter 4 how the stress associated with migration may result in the worsening of existing physical illness, such as cancer, or the development of new physical problems. We have also noted that minority cultural groups may exist in social and economic contexts which are stressful and threatening to their health and general wellbeing. Thus if we consider that new immigrants are often at the bottom of the socioeconomic pile, then they can be seen also to fall victim to many of the other variables described in Table 5.1. For instance, unemployment, poor coping resources, negative life events and small social networks could all be corollaries of 'new immigrant' status. These factors must be kept in mind when examining the more abstract concept of culture in relation to health and disease.

### Dimensions of culture associated with disease

In Chapter 2 we reviewed some large-scale studies of how cultures differ along certain social dimensions. These dimensions had the virtue of being empirically identified (rather than simply being a product of theorizing) and can be related to health inasmuch as the dimensions may relate to the social processes described above. For instance, it has been suggested that cultures which put an emphasis on collectivism have a prophylactic effect on disease because they promote harmony within small supportive groups. This would imply that levels of disease in collectivist cultures are lower than in individualist cultures (see Triandis *et al.*, 1988).

In 1991 Bond, of the Chinese University of Hong Kong, published the results of a study which specifically addressed the relationship between different cultural values and physical health. First of all Bond explored the extent to which people from different countries held certain values to be important. The variation between 23 countries was simplified statistically into two dimensions. The first of these dimensions has 'Social integration' at one pole and 'Cultural inwardness' at the other. Social integration refers to holding values of tolerance towards and harmony with others. This pole also emphasizes patience, non-competitiveness, trustworthiness and persistence. Social integration thus reflects the coming together of peoples, perhaps from different cultures, in an environment which nurtures social relationships. The polar opposite of this is cultural inwardness, which includes values of respect for tradition, a sense of cultural superiority and the observation of rites and social rituals.

The second dimension identified by Bond had 'Reputation' at one pole and 'Morality' as its polar opposite. Here reputation is concerned with protecting your 'face' (in the sense of not losing face), reciprocation of favours and gifts, and the possession of wealth. Morality, on the other hand, is concerned with a sense of righteousness, keeping oneself 'disinterested and pure' and chastity in women. This second dimension could therefore be thought of as a dimension of 'appearing good'–'behaving good'. What is intriguing about Bond's study is that these dimensions, which initially appear rather abstract and hard to grasp, do indeed appear to have relevance to physical diseases.

It is well known that the level of economic development within a country influences the health of its citizens. However, the relationship between Bond's dimensions and disease held up even after the influence of Gross National Product (GNP) per capita was controlled for. It therefore appears that variations in cultural values can account for at least some of the variation in disease prevalence across countries. Furthermore, while these two dimensions could predict the occurrence of a range of diseases in different countries, the dimensions were not themselves associated with life expectancy. In other words, their ability to predict the occurrence of disease is not confounded by variations in average life expectancy in different countries. Let us look at some of these relationships in more detail.

There was a statistically significant association between holding the values of 'social integration' and the increased incidence of cerebrovascular disease, ulcers of the stomach and duodenum, and neoplasms of the stomach, colon, rectum, rectosignoid junction and anus. This array of ailments would suggest that strongly endorsing the values of social integration may, somehow, be particularly deleterious to the functioning of the digestive system. Endorsing the values at the other end of this dimension, 'cultural inwardness', was not significantly related to any of the diseases studied. On the basis of this data it could therefore be argued that 'cultural inwardness' is a healthier outlook than 'social integration'. However, a careful consideration of these findings suggests a more complex situation.

We have already noted suggestions that collectivism could be a health-promoting attribute because it encourages harmony and social support between members of an 'in-group' (for instance, the extended family, work colleagues or neighbours). It seems that individuals living in a collectivist society exhibit these positive behaviours only towards other members of their 'in-group' and not towards other individuals in the society at large. This focuses the therapeutic impact of 'cultural inwardness' at the community level. It is at this level that 'cultural inwardness', through processes such as collectivism, may benefit the health of people. Communities which do not offer social support or foster harmony between their members will strip individuals of an important coping mechanism and the resulting 'cultural isolation' may, somehow, result in a high incidence of cerebrovascular disease and diseases of the digestive system.

This, then, is another argument for allowing different cultural groups to establish a genuine 'sense of community' wherever they are living. Rather than supporting the 'melting pot' notion of different cultures finding a common denominator, Bond's research can thus be interpreted as supporting the integrity of cultural communities as a mechanism for promoting health. However, communities also function in a wider context. In order for communities to provide their potential benefits, the societies in which they live need to be tolerant towards them. In recent years there has been much debate on whether immigrants should locate in areas where their predecessors settled, or whether they should 'integrate' with the nationals of the host country. It would seem that 'cultural inwardness' is the healthiest option in the short term, for the reasons outlined above. In the long term, when immigrants are genuinely accepted as a part of a local community, then they may accrue the same health benefits from such communities as they do from their own 'cultural community'. It would, however, also be important to investigate how the effect of group densities (Halpern, 1993, see Chapter 4) interacts with long- and short-term integration strategies.

Bond's (1991) second dimension, 'Reputation–Morality', was also related to physical health. The 'reputation' end of this dimension was significantly associated with acute myocardial infarction and other ischemic heart disease. It was also, like the other dimension, associated with neoplasms of the colon, rectum, rectosignoid junction and anus. In addition it was associated with neoplasms of the trachea, bronchi and lungs. The influence of the 'reputation' end of this dimension thus seems to be quite pervasive influencing cardiac function, and the digestive and respiratory systems. The opposite end of the dimension, 'morality', was significantly associated with only one disease, cirrhosis of the liver. Taking the two dimensions together, the strongest relationship was with neoplasms of the rectum, rectosignoid junction and anus. However, among the diseases studied by Bond, neither of these dimensions was related to the occurrence of other diseases, such as chronic rheumatic heart disease, atherosclerosis, hypertension and neoplasms of the breast and cervix uteri.

Why statistically significant relationships exist between each dimension and some diseases, but not others, is not clear. It may be that some diseases are more influenced by the psycho-social processes that cultures have an impact on than are others. It may also be that some diseases are influenced by psychosocial or cultural factors which we are as yet unaware of. Clearly much research is needed to clarify such links. From the point of view of our present argument, the point to be taken on board is that cultural variations in values are associated with the occurrence of some diseases. Thus cultural differences are indeed related to physical health.

## ARE SOME CULTURES HEALTHIER THAN OTHERS?

If cultural differences are related to health, this begs the question, 'Are some cultures healthier than others?' The simple answer seems to be 'yes'. Of particular interest here are the Seventh-Day Adventist studies. One of the factors which influences the lifestyle of Seventh-Day Adventists is their belief that the human body is the 'temple' of the Holy Spirit. As such, the body is a sacred place to be treated with respect. You may recall from the introductory chapter of this book, that the word 'culture' derives from the ways in which people seek to 'cultivate' a positive relationship with their God(s). Since different cultures encourage different ways of living, this is another way in which culture can influence physical health.

Seventh-Day Adventists constitute a culture which forms communities throughout the world. Ilola (1990), reviewing studies on Seventh-Day Adventists, states that 'numerous studies from different countries have shown that Seventh-Day Adventists (SDAs) live longer and are healthier than their country-men' (p. 287). The diet of SDAs, based on biblical principles, is based around unrefined foods, grains, vegetable protein, fruits and vegetables. A survey of 40,000 SDAs in the USA found that half were vegetarian, 90 per cent did not consume alcohol, 84 per cent drank less than one cup of coffee per day and 99 per cent did not smoke. Compared with the general population, SDAs appear to have a lower incidence of lung cancer or breast cancer—in fact, cancer of any sort. For those SDAs who do develop cancers, they have better survival rates. Similarly, SDAs have a lower incidence of circulatory diseases. Australian studies have found lower systolic and diastolic blood pressure, lower plasma cholesterol levels and higher lung ventilator capacity in SDAs, compared to the general population. Thus both risk factors and serious diseases appear to be less prevalent in SDA communities than in the general population of their co-nationals.

Ilola also suggests that the degree of adherence to the SDA lifestyle constitutes a 'dose–response' relationship, in that less adherence is associated with greater health risk. The SDA studies illustrate the importance of lifestyle for health. Every culture encourages a particular 'style' of living. When these styles are analysed in terms of the ingestion of foods and other substances, they produce powerful predictors of physical health. Indeed it is through 'consumption customs' that culture, quite literally, 'gets inside of you'.

## CULTURES AND THEIR HEALTH PROBLEMS

It would be wrong to suggest that cultural variations, be it in terms of behaviour, nutrition or other factors, can account for diseases of all kinds. This is certainly not the case. Some diseases are caused by factors quite unrelated to sociocultural processes. Although even here it is worth acknowledging that the way in which such diseases are experienced, expressed and treated, may well be influenced, to some extent at least, by cultural factors. Notwithstanding this important point I would like to review some forms of physical suffering which are found more commonly in certain cultural groups than in others. Black (1989) describes four types of disease categories which are especially relevant to different cultural groups: genetically determined diseases, acquired diseases, diseases which result from the use of indigenous medicines and practices, and diseases related to the poor socioeconomic conditions in which many immigrant groups find themselves. In this section we will consider some examples from the first three of these categories, giving particular emphasis to the first.

## Genetically determined diseases

One hereditary blood disease, sickle-cell anaemia, is so called because the blood cells contain abnormal haemoglobin and when the supply of oxygen is low, these cells, rather than being rounded, adopt the quarter moon shape of a sickle. They are then able to carry less oxygen than the normal rounded blood cells. They also gather together in the blood stream, preventing their passage along capillaries and causing infarction. As a consequence the supply of oxygen to vital organs may be reduced or interrupted. This may result in progressive organ failure and brain damage.

Sickle-cell anaemia is caused by a recessive gene. Thus the majority of people who have this gene are carriers but not sufferers. However, if two people with the recessive gene have a child, then that child will experience sickle-cell anaemia. The sickle-cell gene has a high frequency of occurrence in a number of countries, especially western parts of Africa and southern India. While its high rates of occurrence in the

West Indies and the USA may be historically accounted for by the slave trade, it is also found in the indigenous population of the north coast of the Mediterranean, the Persian Gulf and Saudi Arabia. Thus immigrants from any of these areas will have a 'higher than local average' chance of having or transmitting the disease. Sickle-cell anaemia is, of course, just one of many genetically determined blood diseases which occur with different frequencies across cultural groups. For those involved in diagnosing and treating such diseases a knowledge of these cultural variations is vital.

A second example of a genetically determined disease is lactase deficiency which is brought about by a recessive gene with high penetrance. In other words, although the gene responsible for lactase deficiency is recessive, it usually manages to penetrate into the phenotype; its effects are expressed. The symptoms of lactase deficiency become apparent when an individual consumes milk-based products. In older children (6–7 years and above) and adults the consumption of milk results in abdominal distension, flatulence, abdominal pain or discomfort and occasionally diarrhoea. Although not necessarily a serious condition, it is nonetheless interesting: it is a product, not of genetics alone, but of an interaction between environmental (actually eco-cultural) factors and genetics. I first learnt about lactase deficiency through being told that Chinese people were unable to tolerate a high intake of milk-based products. The rather ethnocentric inference was that 'the rest of us' were. In fact, the great majority of the world's population is 'lactase deficient'.

At birth we are all endowed with intestinal lactase which help us to break down and metabolize our mother's milk. For most people, the amount of lactase produced in their intestine declines to relatively low levels by about the age of 6 or 7. It remains at this lower level from then on. However, for the majority of north, central and western Europeans, and their descendants, as well as some nomadic cultures who depend on the consumption of large amounts of milk from goats or camels, the level of intestinal lactase remains undiminished throughout life. This lactase retention appears to be due to a dominant gene with high penetrance. Once again, because of the genetic basis of lactase intolerance, its incidence varies geographically. People of Chinese descent do indeed appear to have one of the highest levels of lactase intolerance. However, only a minority of these may become symptomatic after drinking, say, a glass of milk. Nonetheless it is important for clinicians to recognize the cultural distribution of this disease and to avoid confusing it with milk allergy.

As a final point on genetically determined conditions, it is important to acknowledge that sometimes these diseases are, in fact, a direct product of cultural practices. For example, among Asian Moslems, marriages between first or second cousins are more common than in other cultures. This practice increases the likelihood of their children falling victim to recessive metabolic disorders and possibly of a child being born malformed. However, it is also very important to emphasize that among such consanguineous marriages the probability of such occurrences is still extremely low.

## Acquired diseases

Nutritional rickets refers to faulty or inadequate bone growth and it has proved to be a particular problem among Asian immigrants to Britain. Black (1989) describes a number of factors contributing to rickets in Asian children: inadequate exposure to sunlight (possibly due to the Moslem custom of covering the arms and legs); strict vegetarian diet (especially for Hindus); use of cow's milk for infant feeding (having little vitamin D); maternal deficiency of vitamin D and a poor uptake of vitamin preparations. The 'Stop Rickets' and 'Asian Mother and Baby' campaigns specifically targeted Asian communities in Britain. These initiatives aimed to create awareness of the role of vitamin D in maintaining good health, with programmes recognizing that each cultural group had to be targeted in a manner which acknowledged differences in their dietary customs, religious beliefs and socioeconomic conditions. Once again, this example of nutritional rickets in immigrant Asian communities illustrates direct links between cultural customs and physical disease. However, these campaigns have also been criticized for problematizing the culture of immigrants, rather than recognizing socioeconomic aspects of rickets as a disease of poverty (see Chapter 8).

## Traditional healing and iatrogenic diseases

Culturally 'traditional' treatments, like many 'modern' treatments developed in industrialized societies, sometimes produce 'side' effects. For some treatments the unwanted effects are as predictable as the 'wanted', or desired, effects. This brief discussion does not therefore suggest that 'traditional' treatments are somehow more 'primitive' because they can produce unhealthy responses in their recipients. Anyone who doubts this need only consult the *British National Formulary* (the BNF, or 'pharmacological bible') to be aware of the huge range, sometimes fatal, of unwanted effects produced by modern medicines. Clinicians should, however, be aware of some of the more common iatrogenic problems which can result from traditional treatments or practices.

In some Asian communities there is a practice of placing black make-up (surma) around the eyes and inside the eyelids in order to prevent infections and for cosmetic effect. This 'make-up' can be made from a variety of substances, one of which is lead sulphide. Over time, with repeated use, dangerous levels of lead may be absorbed through the eye lids. The use of non-lead-based substances for this eye make-up, however, is quite safe.

'Coin rubbing' is a traditional practice common among Vietnamese people. However, coin rubbing can produce lesions on the skin. In some unfortunate cases these marks have been misinterpreted as indications of physical child abuse. Some people of Chinese origin believe that pinching or squeezing either side of the trachea will alleviate persistent coughing. This procedure can produce considerable bruising which might also be misinterpreted.

For another example, recall the 'female circumcision' or 'genital mutilation' described in the first chapter. This is still practised by many peoples throughout the world, including immigrants to more industrialized societies. It can, however, without doubt produce suffering. Beyond the immediate distress which may be experienced, girls can subsequently develop serious medical conditions and find sexual intercourse painful. Nonetheless, it is important to recognize each of the above practices in their cultural context. This does not necessarily mean accepting them. Instead, the clinician will be more successful in changing undesirable practices if he or she can understand them to the extent of being able to offer suggestions for their safe replacement while still retaining some aspect of their cultural function.

## CULTURAL UNDERSTANDINGS OF THE HUMAN BODY

It can be difficult to understand the function of a healing practice without also being aware of the rationale upon which the practice rests. Different understandings of how the human body works should, and do, lead logically to different ways of 'fixing it'. It will therefore be useful to briefly consider some of the different cultural metaphors for understanding the workings of the human body. Perhaps the most widely held view is that which refers to the notion of balance and imbalance in the body. According to this conception the various systems within a healthy body are seen as being in harmony. Imbalance, resulting in illness, can result from physical, psychological, nutritional, environmental or spiritual influences which tip this balance.

The humoral theory is an example of a balance metaphor. This theory was developed into a systematic account of disease by Hippocrates and subsequently elaborated upon by Galen in the second century, spreading throughout the Roman and Arab world. Whether the presence of this theory elsewhere (for instance, throughout Latin America) derives from the same source, or can be accounted for by indigenous beliefs, is unclear. Hippocrates saw the body as being made up of four liquids or humours. These were blood, phlegm, yellow bile and black bile. Too much, or too little, of one of these humours would put the body 'out of balance', resulting in disease. It is also interesting to note that Hippocrates understood these humours to be linked to behaviour. His term 'melancholia' (an excess of black bile) is still in use in today's 'modern' medicine to describe behaviour of depressive affect. His other terms are also in common parlance: sanguine (meaning animated, hopeful or florid, resulting from too much blood), phlegmatic (meaning lethargic or placid, resulting from too much phlegm) and choleric (meaning bad-tempered, resulting from too much yellow bile). Excesses of these humours were treated by bleeding, purging, vomiting and starvation. Deficits were made up through the ingestion of special medicines. Of course, these ideas continue to influence popular thinking in industrialized countries, especially with regard to maintaining an 'optimal' or balanced weight. The bulimic, who vomits or purges in order to retain 'a balance', is a distressing example of this.

In Latin America a common theory of disease relates to the balance between 'hot' and 'cold'. However, this categorization does not refer to temperature as such, but rather to the 'power' intrinsic to different substances. Illness is treated by ingesting substances which counteract an imbalance. Some illnesses are 'hot', others 'cold'. Somebody who is suffering from a 'hot' condition, for example menstruating, would be given 'cold' food only. Another example of the concept of balance is the Chinese notion of the 'yin' and 'yang' forces. Yin has the attributes of darkness, moistness and femininity, while yang is characterized as being bright, hot, dry and masculine. Different organs of the body possess yin and yang in different proportion. For instance, the heart and lungs have an excess of yin, while the stomach and gallbladder have an excess of yang. Illness results from inappropriate combinations of yin and yang at different points of the body's interconnected energy system. One well-known way of treating such an imbalance is through acupuncture.

There are, of course, also other philosophical systems emanating from different cultures which give other accounts for the way our well-being is mediated. However, once again, there is a danger of oversimplifying the relationship between culture and health. Health systems, especially those found in the 'Western' world, reflect many understandings of health. In order to appreciate that 'Western' health care does not have an absolute and definitive approach to understanding illness and well-being, let us briefly consider the work of Rogers (1991).

Rogers described seven metaphorical accounts, found in contemporary 'Western' societies, of how diseases interact with bodily function (see Table 5.2). These metaphors are embraced by different subcultures to varying extents. Whatever metaphor is embraced will have consequences for understanding the cause and treatment of a disease. For instance, the 'body as machine' metaphor welcomes biomedical interventions because they represent the way to 'fix' what is 'broken'. On the other hand, the 'inequality of access' metaphor calls for socioeconomic intervention that will distribute resources more evenly. It is quite common for people to endorse more than one of these metaphors. Professional disputes often arise when metaphors clash and clinicians are intolerant of alternative explanations. Endorsing one metaphor over another usually has resource implications. For example, the 'health promotion' metaphor may call for resources to be channelled into creating healthy lifestyles, while the 'body under siege' metaphor encourages the development of resources for

**Table 5.2:** A summary of Wendy Rogers' (1991) metaphors for health and illness

| Metaphor | Themes related to poor physical health |
|---|---|
| Cultural critique | Inequality, exploitation, disadvantage; modern medicine as an institution of hegemonic power often ineffective in caring or curing, possibly feminism |
| Willpower | Illness as a challenge; power of positive thinking will aid recovery; individual in control rather than social factors, medicine as assistance to own efforts |
| Health promotion | Can be avoided or delayed; due to inappropriate lifestyle, lack of equilibrium, environmental concerns, commercial exploitation, poor eduction |
| Body as machine | Pharmaceuticals critical in 'fixing' dysfunctions; medical excellence through technological expertise; personal responsibility for body maintenance |
| Inequality of access | Injustices between rich and poor; impact of capitalism; health a fundamental human right, modern medicine effective but inequitably distributed because of differences in income, class, education |
| Body under seige | Struggling in a hostile world; germs exploiting emotional distress; not a 'challenge'; conversion of stress into illness; self-denigration, needing help |
| Robust individualism | Stress and pollution of modern life; health a valued investment; self-determination; personal responsibility; consumer selection of expert opinions; health care in the market place |

coping with problems as they arise. This might include the manufacture of vitamins or antidepressants, or the provision of relaxation exercises and rehabilitative services.

In many ways the health professions are health-subcultures, each endorsing certain metaphors over others and therefore understanding the relationship between health and disease in different ways. Within each professional subculture, as within each social group or culture, there is, of course, great variation. However, seeing different health professions as different 'cultures', which work through different 'communities', may help us to understand the interprofessional rivalry which can be a feature of multidisciplinary work. This organizational interpretation of the link between cultures, communities and health, while intriguing, is at a tangent to the purpose of this chapter. We therefore return to consider disease and 'culture'.

## CULTURE AND REACTION TO DISEASES

When people from different cultures suffer with the same disease they naturally will use different terms to describe it, because their languages are different. However, even when the same language is used, in the same country, confusion can still arise. Ilola (1990) describes a young physician, trained in a metropolitan centre, but undertaking an internship in rural Tennessee, USA. There he encountered 'sick-as-hell anaemia', 'very close veins' and 'smiling mighty Jesus' (spinal meningitis)! In this section we look at how cultures understand the same illness in different ways. In essence, human suffering is explained by different cultures in different ways. The form of explanation may reflect the projection of a culture's values into the experience of suffering. In the following sections we review cultural perspectives on pain, deafness and AIDS. While there is a large literature on cultural aspects of many physical conditions, I have chosen these three for specific reasons. Pain is a problem common to most physical conditions which cause suffering. Pain is often the 'signal' that something is wrong and so, as a 'medium' of communication, it is important to understand pain in a cultural context. We review research on deafness, taking it to be one example of a physical disability. Deafness was specifically chosen because many people would assume that its cause is so 'obvious' that it cannot be influenced by cultural factors. The third condition, HIV/AIDS, is focused on because of the frightening impact which this virus has had on so many cultures, because it appears to be more of a problem in some cultural minority groups than in others and because of the racist assumptions which have characterized the search for its source. Each of these conditions can now routinely be encountered by community clinicians working across the cultures of our inner cities.

## Pain

Here again we encounter the warning to refrain from simplistic stereotyping of cultural groups, this time with regard to people's experience of pain:

> . . . everyone has a cultural heritage which is part and parcel of an individual's health practices. The practical answer is not to learn in detail the infinite varieties of culture but to be aware of these varieties and how they might affect one's health practices. I am totally opposed to training anyone in the details of a particular ethnic group, for this will ultimately squeeze people into unreal categories, and 'typecast' their culture just as we have rigidified diagnoses. What I favour is making practitioners sensitive to the patient's heritage, their own heritage, and to what happens when different heritages come together.
>
> (Zola, 1983, p. 227).

Over the last 30 years there have been a good number of investigations into the interplay between culture and pain experience. However, differences in methodology have made the results hard to integrate, although generally it is believed

that culture does influence pain experiences and/or pain behaviour. To delineate more clearly the relationships between
culture and pain, Lipton and Marbach (1984) studied consecu-
tive referrals to a facial pain clinic in New York. They ran-
domly selected 50 patients from each of five prominent
groups in the hospital's catchment area (Black, Irish, Italian,
Jewish or Puerto Rican). Note that these categories reflect potentially overlapping criteria of colour, religion and geo-
graphy, regarding culture (presumably Black Italian Jews
were screened out of the study!).

The pain patients completed a comprehensive questionnaire
concerning the physical experience of pain, its cognitive and
emotional aspects, how it interferes with daily functioning,
and the patient's health-seeking behaviour. Regardless of ethnicity these patients gave equivalent responses for two-thirds
of the items on the questionnaire. They did not, for instance,
differ in the degree to which they experienced their pain as
stabbing or sharp, or in the extent to which they worried
about their pain. Each group gave equal importance to seeing
pain as a warning that something was wrong and described
themselves as being able to take pain equally well. The majority of patients from each group claimed that they never cried
or moaned (!) about their face pain, while an equivalent number of patients from each group claimed that they would not
worry about having an operation as long as it cured their
facial pain. Thus differences in culture did not extend to influencing these pain patients on the majority of items.

Nonetheless, of equal interest are those items on which there
were cultural differences. We have already noted that cultural
groups live in a variety of socioeconomic conditions and that
these conditions can influence health. Lipton and Marbach
therefore investigated a range of factors, which they believed
were not intrinsic attributes of different cultural groups, but
which might differ between different groups and so make it
appear that cultural differences existed, when in fact they did
not. The results of this investigation are fascinating in

themselves. Table 5.3 shows the results. Patients attending the clinic from each cultural group differed significantly in their average age, in the ratio of males to females, in their income and education, in the proportion who identified themselves as 'American' and in the proportion who were third generation, or more, born in the USA.

The cultural groups did not only differ on social and demographic variables, they also differed significantly on psychologically more immediate measures. These included social assimilation, medical acculturation, psychological distress and symptom history. The term 'social assimilation' describes the extent to which a minority culture group member has integrated into the dominant culture, for instance, by having close or intimate relationships outside their cultural group. The degree of ethnocentricity, friendship solidarity within one's own group and the strength of family traditions, each differed significantly across the five cultural groups. 'Medical acculturation' refers to the exchange of cultural health norms for the biomedical norms of the 'mainstream' United States culture. The extent of biomedical health knowledge, of scepticism about it and of the adoption of a dependency role when sick, all differed across cultural groups. Puerto Rican patients reported the highest levels of psychological distress and Irish patients the lowest levels. There were also significant differences across the five ethnic groups in the reported chronicity of pain, the occurrence of other pain, the number of medical doctors previously consulted, the number of different treatments sought, and even diagnosis given. In contrast to the previously noted difference between Puerto Rican and Irish patients' psychological symptoms, they were both more likely to be given a diagnosis of Temporomandibular Joint Syndrome (TMJS) than were black patients.

These variables therefore represent a broad spectrum of life experiences and all varied across the five cultural groups studied by Lipton and Marbach. It is little wonder that the provision of multicultural health services is so complex, as there are many aspects of health which could be influenced by the above differences. For example, with regard to the pain clinic patients, these 'confounding variables' accounted for apparent cultural differences in reported fear of cancer, ability to enjoy oneself, belief that 'I probably deserve this pain . . .', attending a medical doctor once pain is experienced and willingness to take medication to alleviate suffering. It is, therefore, not only the cultural differences between groups *per se* that influence health, but also differences between them arising from the different contexts in which they exist.

What then of the 'pure' cultural differences in pain? Culture did account for differences in the extent to which pain was experienced as a 'dull ache', or as 'very severe, almost unbearable'. There were also significant differences in the extent to which patients wondered about what they had done to have the pain, in their feeling that they might 'lose control', about the benefit of complaining and the importance of trying to hide pain. Likelihood of becoming emotional when describing the pain and desire to have other people around when experiencing pain, also differed. Finally, whether the pain affected appetite, the ability to work and the likelihood of having been to many medical doctors, were also influenced by cultural group membership.

The most compelling finding to come out of Lipton and Marbach's research is not, however, about the similarities or differences across cultural groups in their experience of pain or their pain behaviour; instead it is that each cultural group appeared to have different 'triggers' for their pain experience. Different factors appear to be associated with pain in each cultural group. In the case of Black patients, the greater their degree of dependency (during sickness) on 'lay' social/ cultural group members, the greater was their emotional and expressive response to pain, and the greater was their disturbance in daily functioning. For Irish patients, longstanding close relationships ('friendship solidarity') with other ethnic Irish was related to greater reporting of disruption in daily

**Table 5.3:** Descriptive data for different cultural groups in a study of pain experience

| Independent variable | Ethnic group | | | | | | | | | | F-ratio |
|---|---|---|---|---|---|---|---|---|---|---|---|
| | Black | | Irish | | Italian | | Jewish | | Puerto Rican | | |
| | X | SD | X | SD | X | SD | X | SD | X | SD | |
| *Sociodemographic* | | | | | | | | | | | |
| Age (in years) | 47.2 | 18.4 | 36.2 | 15.6 | 33.7 | 13.3 | 42.2 | 17.2 | 36.4 | 11.4 | 6.42† |
| Sex (% male) | 25.0 | 43.7 | 0 | 0 | 9.1 | 29.0 | 18.9 | 39.5 | 37.5 | 48.9 | 7.71† |
| Position (% youngest and middle) | 60.0 | 49.5 | 71.4 | 45.7 | 54.5 | 50.3 | 66.0 | 47.8 | 68.7 | 46.8 | 0.99† |
| Income (% greater than $18,000) | 30.0 | 46.3 | 73.3 | 44.7 | 71.4 | 45.6 | 50.9 | 50.5 | 31.2 | 46.8 | 9.79† |
| Education (years completed) | 11.0 | 4.1 | 13.1 | 2.6 | 12.8 | 2.2 | 13.5 | 2.6 | 11.2 | 2.2 | 8.29† |
| Generation American (% third or more) | 85.0 | 36.1 | 73.3 | 44.7 | 45.4 | 50.2 | 41.5 | 49.7 | 6.2 | 24.4 | 26.27† |
| Ethnic identification (% 'American') | 55.0 | 50.2 | 26.7 | 44.7 | 45.4 | 50.3 | 71.7 | 45.5 | 12.5 | 33.4 | 13.49† |
| *Social assimilation* (score on index) (higher score indicates greater degree of acculturation) | | | | | | | | | | | |
| Ethnic exclusivity | 1.10 | 0.54 | 1.73 | 0.45 | 1.64 | 0.57 | 1.31 | 0.58 | 1.25 | 0.56 | 12.15† |
| Friendship solidarity | 2.60 | 1.44 | 3.00 | 0.85 | 2.48 | 0.97 | 2.64 | 1.09 | 1.53 | 1.32 | 10.44† |
| Family tradition | 1.44 | 1.18 | 1.85 | 1.11 | 2.15 | 0.97 | 1.84 | 0.99 | 1.33 | 1.20 | 4.25† |

| | | | | | | | | | | | |
|---|---|---|---|---|---|---|---|---|---|---|---|
| *Medical acculturation* (score on index) (higher score indicates greater degree of acculturation) | | | | | | | | | | | |
| Scepticism | 0.70 | 0.91 | 1.33 | 0.71 | 1.09 | 0.91 | 0.88 | 0.89 | 1.19 | 0.81 | 4.32† |
| Dependency | 1.00 | 0.78 | 1.33 | 0.80 | 1.27 | 0.62 | 1.26 | 0.68 | 0.94 | 0.66 | 3.17† |
| Health knowledge | 5.90 | 3.14 | 5.87 | 2.47 | 5.73 | 2.51 | 6.72 | 2.98 | 4.37 | 2.83 | 4.62† |
| *Level of psychological distress* (score on index) | 4.35 | 4.71 | 3.13 | 4.11 | 5.52 | 4.27 | 5.72 | 3.82 | 6.73 | 4.22 | 5.19† |
| *Symptom and treatment history* | | | | | | | | | | | |
| Duration (% chronic) | 35.0 | 48.2 | 60.0 | 49.5 | 72.7 | 45.0 | 69.8 | 46.3 | 75.0 | 43.7 | 6.23† |
| Other pain (% none) | 35.0 | 48.2 | 73.3 | 44.7 | 55.0 | 50.3 | 34.5 | 48.0 | 43.7 | 50.1 | 5.65† |
| Change in location of pain (% no change) | 45.0 | 50.2 | 41.7 | 50.0 | 41.2 | 49.9 | 56.2 | 50.1 | 56.2 | 50.1 | 1.04 |
| Pain severity | 70.0 | 31.5 | 61.7 | 31.8 | 62.5 | 31.2 | 63.7 | 29.7 | 54.7 | 29.9 | 1.57 |
| Number doctors previously consulted (% seeing 3 or more) | 25.0 | 43.7 | 66.7 | 47.6 | 59.1 | 49.7 | 56.6 | 50.0 | 25.0 | 43.7 | 8.99† |
| Number different treatments previously received (% 2 or more) | 20.0 | 40.4 | 53.3 | 50.4 | 50.0 | 50.5 | 32.1 | 47.1 | 0 | 0 | 13.47† |
| Diagnosis (% TMJS) | 50.0 | 50.5 | 73.3 | 44.7 | 68.2 | 47.0 | 66.0 | 47.8 | 81.2 | 39.4 | 3.12* |

* Significant, $p < 0.05$; † significant, $p < 0.01$.

Reproduced from Lipton and Marbach (1984) with kind permission from Elsevier Science Ltd, The Boulevard, Langford Lane, Kidlington OX5 1GB.

functioning and a non-emotionally expressive response to their pain. Italian patients' response to pain was best predicted by the length of time they had the pain. Chronic pain (for at least six months) was associated with both an emotional and an expressive response, as well as a disruption in performing physical activities. The level of reported psychological distress was most important for explaining the pain of Jewish patients because a high level of distress was strongly associated with an emotionally expressive pain response and with interference in daily functioning. Finally, for Puerto Rican patients, high psychological distress, strong 'friendship solidarity', and dependency on other Puerto Ricans when sick and suffering chronic pain were all associated with an emotionally expressive pain response and significant disruption in daily activities attributable to pain.

Overall this research suggests that while cultural groups may report similar responses to pain, different factors influence their responses. Different cultures present different settings and conditions for the expression of pain. Nonetheless, we should not expect all Irish, or all Italians or all Blacks to be equally influenced by intracultural factors. Lipton and Marbach's research does, however, help us to understand how, within different cultural groups, individuals are influenced by particular psychosocial processes. A very practical clinical example of this would be that not all cultures are equally willing to use 'pain killing' medication. Poliakoff (1993) suggests that many Chinese people fear that such medication may give them a feeling of being out of control. In addition to this, some Chinese people also have a belief that pain killers cause sweating and that this loss of body fluid will induce weakness.

People of particular faiths may accept pain as their due. For instance, Hindus who believe they are facing death may wish to do so 'clear headed' rather than sedated. Negative feelings, such as pain, may be attributed to wrongs which they have committed in the past. Thus the reluctance of some patients to accept analgesics may have no relationship to the severity of their pain experience, but instead be to do with the extent to which psychosocial factors, particular to their own culture, impact upon them as individuals. This level of analysis moves us beyond the stereotypical 'one culture–one type of person' perspective to a 'one culture–several salient psychosocial processes which individuals will encounter' perspective. This is a much more sensitive and realistic level of analysis. It recognizes the dynamic between the individual and his or her social context—that the will of the individual, and the 'grain' of his or her cultural setting, each contribute to the person's behaviour. While it is more sensitive to the realism of clinical practice, we must also acknowledge that it allows for less specificity and predictability. We cannot say with certainty that because Simon is Jewish and experiencing facial pain, and because he reports a high level of psychological distress, that he will necessarily also report significant disruption in performing his usual activities. We can, however, say that this would usually be the case for a member of the Jewish culture in the USA. The fact that he may not adhere to this relationship may be very significant, not only in understanding him as a person, but also in providing an effective intervention to help him.

## Deafness

Hearing loss is one of the commonest health problems in industrialized societies. People suffering from loss of hearing are often stigmatized. For instance, problems in communication are often attributed to the person suffering hearing loss being rude, uninterested or stupid. One of the major causes of hearing loss appears to be working in a noisy environment. Migrant workers are often over-represented in noisy industries such as manufacturing or construction. Even when companies do provide ear protection and information leaflets on the importance of avoiding loud noises, employees often continue to expose themselves to potentially harmful levels of

**Table 5.4:** Causal attributions for deafness

| Attribution | Community attribution score* (rank in brackets) | | | | | | $F†$ | $p$ |
|---|---|---|---|---|---|---|---|---|
| | Anglo | German | Italian | Greek | Chinese | Arabic | | |
| Ageing | (1)3.06 | (2)2.68‡ | (1)2.83 | (2)2.75‡ | (1)2.75‡ | (2)2.61‡ | 3.15 | <0.01 |
| Industrial noise | (2)2.99 | (1)2.71‡ | (2)2.69 | (1)2.82‡ | (5)2.42‡ | (4)2.45‡ | 9.21 | <0.0001 |
| Heredity | (3)2.74 | (5)2.38‡ | (6½)2.26‡ | (7)2.28‡ | (6)2.34‡ | (10)2.10‡ | 10.33 | <0.0001 |
| Loud music | (4)2.70 | (4)2.50 | (6½)2.26‡ | (5)2.31‡ | (7)2.32‡ | (13)1.87‡ | 8.99 | <0.0001 |
| Chance, could happen to anyone | (5)2.55 | (3)2.57 | (3)2.50 | (3)2.53 | (3½)2.43 | (6½)2.25 | 1.54 | >0.05 |
| Past injuries | (6)2.41 | (6½)2.23 | (5)2.38 | (8)2.27 | (3½)2.43 | (5)2.42 | 1.30 | <0.01 |
| Infectious germs | (7)2.10 | (6½)2.23 | (8)2.13 | (6)2.29 | (2)2.52‡ | (3)2.57‡ | 5.61 | <0.0001 |
| Person's temperament (doesn't bother listening) | (8½)1.87 | (11)1.78 | (11½)1.85 | (11)1.95 | (15)1.70 | (15)1.72 | 1.47 | >0.05 |
| Stress and tension | (8½)1.87 | (8)2.16‡ | (10)1.86 | (9)2.13‡ | (12½)1.74 | (11)1.97 | 3.83 | <0.01 |
| Person in poor health, 'run down' | (10)1.82 | (9)1.94 | (13)1.78 | (13)1.92 | (8)2.24‡ | (12)1.94 | 5.60 | <0.0001 |
| Drugs | (11)1.81 | (10)1.81 | (9)2.00 | (13)1.92 | (11)1.75 | (16)1.67 | 2.07 | >0.05 |
| Poor medical care | (12)1.73 | (12)1.64 | (11½)1.85 | (10)1.96‡ | (9)2.04‡ | (9)2.15‡ | 5.44 | <0.001 |
| God's will | (13)1.52 | (14)1.49 | (4)2.43‡ | (4)2.46‡ | (10)1.81‡ | (1)3.09‡ | 50.16 | <0.0001 |
| Upsetting or disturbing event | (14)1.49 | (13)1.54 | (14)1.75‡ | (15)1.81‡ | (12½)1.74‡ | (6½)2.25‡ | 10.48 | <0.0001 |
| Poor diet | (15)1.39 | (15)1.45 | (17)1.43 | (17)1.43 | (16)1.69‡ | (18)1.45 | 3.39 | <0.01 |
| Karma | (16)1.13 | (16)1.24 | (18)1.25 | (18)1.32‡ | (14)1.72‡ | (17)1.63‡ | 15.62 | <0.0001 |
| Person's bad actions, sins | (17)1.09 | (18)1.09 | (16)1.53‡ | (16)1.58‡ | (17)1.65‡ | (14)1.77‡ | 19.04 | <0.0001 |
| Evil influences e.g. evil eye curse | (18)1.07 | (17)1.10 | (15)1.64‡ | (13)1.92‡ | (18)1.58‡ | (8)2.24‡ | 41.13 | <0.0001 |

* Scores ranged from 4 (almost always explanation) to 1 (rarely).
† df ranged from 5/654 to 5/585.
‡ $t$ contrast between Anglo and other cultural groups' scores yielded $p < 0.01$.
Reproduced from Westbrook *et al.* (1994) with permission. © 1994 Harwood Academic Publishers.

noise. Migrants may be at a particular disadvantage if they are not proficient in the language of the health promotion literature provided by the company. However, a more pervasive problem may be that migrant workers have different 'explanatory models' for deafness.

Westbrook and her colleagues (1994) at the University of Sydney have conducted a series of studies on disability within a multicultural society. They have looked at the causal attributions for mid-life deafness among the Anglo, Chinese, German, Greek, Italian and Arabic communities. The subjects for the study were 665 community health practitioners who were members of each of the above cultural groups. These included medical practitioners, nurses, dentists, physiotherapists, occupational therapists, speech therapists, social welfare and community health workers. These practitioners completed a questionnaire which gave 18 different potential causes for hearing loss in a 35-year-old man. The practitioners rated each cause in terms of how they believed members of their own cultural community would explain hearing loss. They were not giving their own personal ratings. Table 5.4 summarizes the results of the study.

Two audiologists independently rated the likelihood of each of the attributions in Table 5.4 as being the most probable cause of hearing loss. They each agreed that industrial noise, followed by drugs and past injuries would 'often' be cited as the cause of the patient's hearing loss, and that infection, heredity, loud music and poor medical care could 'sometimes' be the cause. As can be seen from the table, none of the ratings from any ethnic group agreed with the ratings of these two specialists. Analysis of variance showed that there was a significant difference across the six ethnic groups for every one of the 18 possible attributions. 'God's will' was the cause over which there was greatest disagreement. It was predicted that the Arabic community would give this top ranking, the Greek and Italian communities would rank it fourth and the Chinese, Anglo and German communities would rank it tenth, thirteenth and fourteenth respectively. It was predicted that the 'ageing' explanation would be rated either the first or second most likely cause by all the cultures.

Another way of looking at this data is by considering whether the top rated attributions were endorsed by the audiologists. Across the six cultures the top eight attributions included the following explanations, not endorsed by the audiologists: chance (all cultures), God's will (Italian, Greek and Arabic), stress and tension (German and Anglo), person's temperament (Anglo), poor health (Chinese), upsetting event and evil eye (Arabic). It is clear that each culture would have a distinct profile for the probable causes of hearing loss, and that they would all differ from the specialists' opinion. This sort of research is especially useful to the community clinician because it emphasizes how he or she may need to act as a go-between for members of minority cultural groups and clinicians in the 'mainstream' centralized health services. This research also points to a problem with health promotion. For if the 'official' line on what causes deafness is different from that which you have been brought up to believe, adopting health-promoting behaviour may also involve a rejection of your own cultural values. This issue will be dealt with in more detail in Chapter 8.

We have emphasized cultural differences with regard to specific diseases. As shown, there are real and significant variations in how people from different cultures explain the cause of deafness. In a related study, Westbrook et al. (1993) investigated the degree of stigma attached to 20 different diseases and disabilities, across the six cultural groups already mentioned. They found a remarkably consistent pattern across all cultural communities: people with asthma, diabetes, heart disease and arthritis were the least stigmatized, while those with AIDS, mental retardation, psychiatric illness and cerebral palsy were the most stigmatized. Comparing their own research with research over the last 23 years, these findings appear remarkably consistent across time also. While AIDS has not previously been included in such studies, it was the most stigmatized condition across all the cultures.

## AIDS/HIV

The human immunosuppression virus (HIV) is one of the most devastating diseases of our time. It is known and experienced throughout the world. It is perhaps the clearest exemplar of the interplay between cultures, communities and health. It has given rise to paranoid reactions towards 'gay communities', drug users, immigrants, haemophiliacs and cultural minorities. It is a fatal disease contracted through specific activities such as sexual intercourse involving the exchange of bodily fluids, the sharing of intravenous needles and blood transfusions. One of the sources of the racism which characterizes reactions to this disease is the suggestion that behaviours, such as sexual intercourse and sharing of needles, occur with significantly greater frequency in some cultural groups than in others. Furthermore, this is probably true.

The World Health Organization gave the following figures for AIDS cases reported up to 30 June 1994: Europe, 115,668; the Americas, 523,777; Africa, 331,376; Asia 8,968; and Oceania (Australia and New Zealand), 5,330. Taking the populations of these continents into account, these figures reflect a huge variation in the prevalence of AIDS cases. For example, in Europe, France with a population of 56 million has reported 30,003 cases, while Germany with a population of 79 million has reported 11,179 cases. While differences in the reporting of cases, as opposed to their actual occurrence, may account for some of the differences observed between countries, it is clear that significant differences do exist. Equally there are significant differences regarding the number of people who are estimated to be HIV positive but who have not yet developed symptoms of AIDS. In this section we firstly consider the impact which AIDS has had on Hispanic communities in the USA. Then we focus on the racist pursuit for the origin of AIDS. These two cases offer an important perspective on *the process through which* we respond to disease in a multicultural society.

### AIDS in Hispanic communities in the USA

In 1994 the USA had the highest number of reported AIDS cases of any country in the world. In fact with 411,907 cases reported by June 1994, the USA not only had more cases than any other country, it also had more reported cases than any continent, including Africa. Singer and her colleagues (1990) from the Hispanic Health Council, Hartford, Connecticut, have given a detailed account of the Hispanic AIDS crisis in the USA. While the Hispanic community constitutes 8 per cent of the population, it accounted for 15 per cent of AIDS cases reported in the USA in 1988. More recent accounts of AIDS confirm its high prevalence among cultural minorities both in the USA and in other industrialized countries. Initially the medical model of the disease focused attention on the individual, rather than on cultural variables and the social, economic and political reality of marginalized communities. Now these realities are being addressed.

Hispanic communities in the USA are not homogeneous. Nonetheless, when statistical averages are compared, for example, to White communities, they live in significantly more poverty and are less well educated. They suffer disproportionately more infectious and parasitic diseases, higher rates of infant mortality and lower life expectancy. Research conducted in the late 1980s found that the rate of HIV infection in Hispanic communities was almost twice as high as that in non-Hispanic communities. Furthermore, the ways in which AIDS is contracted also appears to be different across cultural groups. Table 5.5 gives a breakdown of 'exposure category', or route of contraction, by culture. It is clear from these figures that male homosexual or bisexual contact accounts for a much greater percentage of cases among White, Asian and Pacific Island communities than it does among Hispanic, Native American and Black communities.

**Table 5.5:** Cumulative incidence of AIDS cases through April 1989, United States: percentage of adult/adolescent cases in each exposure category by culture

| Exposure category | Hispanic (%) | White (%) | Black (%) | Asian/ Pac. Isl. (%) | Native Amer. (%) | Total (%) |
|---|---|---|---|---|---|---|
| Male homosexual/ bisexual contact | 42 | 77 | 37 | 75 | 51 | 61 |
| Intravenous drug use (heterosexual- male and female) | 40 | 7 | 38 | 4 | 16 | 20 |
| Male homosexual/ bisexual contact and intravenous drug use | 7 | 7 | 7 | 1 | 14 | 7 |
| Hemophilia/ coagulation disorder | 0.5 | 1 | 0 | 2 | 6 | 1 |
| Heterosexual contact | 5 | 2 | 11 | 3 | 6 | 4 |
| Receipt of blood products or tissue | 1 | 3 | 1 | 8 | 3 | 2 |
| Other/undetermined | 5 | 2 | 5 | 7 | 5 | 3 |

Reproduced from Singer *et al.* (1990) by permission of the American Anthropological Association from *Medical Anthropology Quarterly*, 4:1, March 1990. Not for further reproduction.

Likewise there is a dramatic difference across the cultural groups in the extent to which intravenous drug use has been a route of contracting HIV. Comparisons such as these attest to the degree to which culture, through a variety of social processes and social disadvantages, is pathoplastic (shapes the development) in physical diseases.

Table 5.6 breaks down different possible preventative activities with regard to AIDS undertaken by Hispanic, African or White

Americans. Table 5.7 shows variations in sexual practices across these groups. In both cases there are significant differences between the three groups. Interventions which seek to promote low risk AIDS behaviours need to take into account the reasons for such differences and to build them into prevention programmes. For instance, the traditional cultural stereotypes of male *machismo* (being authoritarian within the family, having extramarital sex, drinking heavily, physically abusing family members, etc.) and of female *marianismo* (women being chaste before marriage, submitting to their husbands' authority, enduring suffering, being morally and spiritually pure, etc.) could easily be seen as providing a context for transmission of HIV through 'hot blooded' Hispanic men chasing Hispanic women. However, heterosexual contact may account for only about 5 per cent of cases, while intravenous drug use and homosexual contact may each account for over 40 per cent of cases. Accurate empirical research on salient issues will help us to understand different perceptions of AIDS; different routes of transmission; the differing length of time between contraction of HIV and the expression of AIDS symptoms; the different propensities towards preventative measures and the different resources which can be brought to bear, all varying across cultural communities.

**Table 5.6:** Reported preventive activities during the previous 12 months: percentage of affirmative responses for each cultural group

|  | Latino | African American | White | All |
|---|---|---|---|---|
| Discussed AIDS-<br>preventive behaviour<br>with sex partner | 35 | 49 | 65 | 47 |
| Avoided sex with<br>prostitutes | 62 | 90 | 84 | 78 |
| Limited number of sex<br>partners | 74 | 85 | 84 | 81 |
| Used condoms more<br>frequently | 34 | 43 | 36 | 38 |

Reproduced from Singer *et al.* (1990) by permission of the American Anthropological Association from *Medical Anthropology Quarterly*, 4:1, March 1990. Not for further reproduction.

**Table 5.7:** Sexual practices and condom use in the past year: percentage of affirmation responses for each cultural group

|  | Latino (*n* = 117) | African Am. (*n* = 100) | White (*n* = 73) | All (*n* = 290) |
|---|---|---|---|---|
| Vaginal intercourse with condoms | 37 | 54 | 33 | 42 |
| Vaginal intercourse without condoms | 69 | 81 | 86 | 78 |
| Anal intercourse without condoms | 17 | 16 | 28 | 19 |
| Oral sex without condoms | 28 | 53 | 67 | 46 |
| Oral sex with condoms | 11 | 20 | 20 | 16 |

Reproduced from Singer *et al.* (1990) by permission of the American Anthropological Association from *Medical Anthropology Quarterly*, 4:1, March 1990. Not for further reproduction.

## AIDS, Africans and racism

Describing the cultural or racial aspect of a disease can be a tricky business. Focusing on the differences between cultural groups can, whether intentionally or otherwise, promote racism, ignorance or naivety. Such allegations are usually made when it is felt that one culture, or cultural group, is being negatively compared with another. But such comparisons, while not necessary, are nonetheless inevitable. If a disease is found more often in one cultural group than in another, it is reasonable for people to ask why and how this should be. However, the ascribing of disease origin to a particular culture, which is then understood to have infected other peoples, is a potentially explosive situation. From a social psychological standpoint the search for an origin or source of disease can take on the function of scapegoating certain social groups or nations. In the case of AIDS, some have argued that the fear aroused by the disease has compelled people to project its source into things which they also fear and/or denigrate. The unspoken rationale goes something like this: 'What is different is dangerous and things which are different from us and dangerous to us, go together.' This sort of 'witch hunt' can certainly be fuelled by the popular media, but, in the case of AIDS, scientists and clinicians have also been caught up in, and become a key part of, the process. While 'we are all human' it is necessary to be aware that the collective forces of 'inhumanity' can draw in clinicians too.

In their book *AIDS, Africa and Racism*, Chirimuuta and Chirimuuta (1989) catalogue explicit examples of racism in ascribing the source of the AIDS epidemic to people of African origin:

> The widespread, uncritical acceptance of the AIDS from Africa hypothesis by the normally sceptical scientific community is most disturbing. It would be comforting to believe that this was a simple mistake or an unfortunate result of an excess of enthusiasm. It seems to us far more likely that the AIDS researchers, the medical 'experts', the media and the public at large are affected by the insidious and frequently unrecognised disease of racism. (p. 136).

How many times have you heard people (perhaps including yourself) say that 'research suggests AIDS started in Africa'? The Chirimuutas' point is that there is good evidence to suggest that this may not be the case and that, regardless of its origin, African peoples are seen as a more fertile 'culture' in which the virus can 'grow'.

When AIDS first appeared in white male American homosexuals, they became obvious scapegoats. However, the Chirimuutas argue, this meant that the disease was still American. Another source was desirable:

> Given the racist stereotyping of black people as dirty, disease carrying and sexually promiscuous it was virtually inevitable that black people, on the first sight of the disease

among them, would be attributed with its source . . .
Racism, not science, motivated the search for the origin of
AIDS. (p. 128).

By 1982, 700 cases of AIDS had been reported in the United
States. Thirty-four of these were Haitian immigrants. Haiti is a
small island off the Florida coast mainly inhabited by the
descendants of African slaves. On the basis of these statistics
it was quickly suggested that gay American tourists visiting
Haiti had contracted the disease from the Haitians. These
American tourists had then passed on the disease to other
Americans (generally homosexuals) on their return to the
USA.

This notion, generated by statistics and derived from 'scientific speculation', was zealously promoted by the American
media gelling together the idea of 'AIDS' with the idea of
'Haitian'. The result was that Haitians resident in the USA
were sacked from their jobs, evicted from their homes and
Haitian prisoners were quarantined. Fortunately, within a
few years, the idea that one country (Haiti) was responsible
for the suffering of another country (USA) did not hold up to
closer scrutiny. It transpired that while there did appear to be
a link between Haiti and the USA, it was in the opposite
direction. Apparently it was the Americans who had brought
AIDS to Haiti and not the other way round. . . . The search for
the 'true' source of AIDS shifted again, this time to the 'dark
continent'.

With the Haitian hypothesis debunked the 'steaming jungles'
deep within the 'hidden interior' of central Africa presented
fertile ground to search for the source of AIDS. Research scientists jetted in, swooping down from the skies, to collect
precious blood samples, swiftly returning to their technological lairs 'back home' for analysis. One of the notions which
arose from this flurry of activity was the 'monkey hypothesis'.
This was the idea that monkeys had transmitted an AIDS-like
virus to humans when Africans were bitten by them, ate

them, gave their children dead monkeys as pets, injected monkey blood as a sexual stimulant or, as I have heard on more than one occasion, 'had sex with a monkey'! What could distance the 'Western world' more from the cause of AIDS than it coming from a monkey in Africa committing an 'unnatural act' with somebody deep in the centre of that disease-ridden continent?

The tragedy of AIDS illustrates the often complex interplay between culture and disease. It is a world-wide scourge; it does show different rates of prevalence across ethnic groups, it is transmitted through specific behaviour patterns and it is so 'bad' that there is a strong desire to 'externalize' its cause and project our fears and anger onto an identifiable target. This way of dealing with a fearful disease is not new. For instance, in the middle ages the English ascribed syphilis to the French. Later the French described it as the 'Italian disease'. There will surely be future epidemics onto which society will graft its racial insecurities. The challenge for clinicians is to be aware of the extent to which they, their colleagues or leading 'authorities' are caught up in their culture's way of dealing with such threats. A key element in being able to do this is understanding the sociocultural symbolism and the function of explaining a disease in one particular way as compared to another.

## RACIAL HYGIENE AND ETHNIC CLEANSING

Culture is intimately related to physical health and disease. We have largely focused on how this interplay can be developed for the good of all peoples. However, we have also noted cultural 'scapegoating' with regard to AIDS/HIV. Perhaps the most horrific example of the destructive interplay between culture and medicine was the 'racial hygiene' practised by the Nazis in the Second World War. Proctor (1988) describes the ethos of racial hygiene as initially promoting the benefits, for all races, of encouraging breeding within well-

educated civilized families, but controlling it among criminals, illiterates and the insane. This ethos then developed into
suggestions that medical care should not be given to the
'weak' since it might encourage the continuation of 'weak'
genes in the racial gene pool. Diseases such as tuberculosis
and leprosy were described as 'our racial friends' because
they attacked and 'weeded out' the weak.

When the Nazis came to power in Germany in the 1930s they
promoted the goal of achieving 'purity' of the Aryan race.
Genetic Courts ruled on what sorts of people should be ster-
ilized. This philosophy of racial purity extended to racial
superiority, culminating in the mass murder of millions of
people who were judged to be of 'inferior race', such as
Gypsies and Jews.

The holocaust is a haunting example of how one culture, the
Nazi culture, saw the relationship between illness and culture, and how it was dealt with. The 'ethnic cleansing' in the
former Yugoslavia, and in and around Ruanda, are poignant
reminders that horrific ways of dealing with cultural differences cannot be dismissed into history, but that they are
part of our present and will undoubtedly be part of our future
too. Without a serious commitment to multiculturalism and
tolerance of different ways of understanding human health
and suffering, clinicians will not be well equipped to prevent
humanity from picking away at, and reopening, its horrific
racist wounds.

## GUIDELINES FOR PROFESSIONAL PRACTICE

1. Clinicians should be aware that the relationship between
   psychosocial stress and health is complex and often in-
   direct. Psychosocial factors can influence health through
   at least three pathways: producing physiological hyperactivity, exacerbating existing disease and reducing
   the body's immunocompetence. Stressful psychosocial

experiences should therefore be addressed in any treatment plan, even when the clinician does not see them as directly related to the presenting complaint. At the very least, such experiences may reduce the beneficial potential of treatment interventions.

2. Cultural differences, the experience of migration or the experience of being a member of a minority group can produce psychosocial stressors which have been shown to influence physical health. Such experiences should therefore be considered risk factors in themselves. Thus even when these experiences are shrugged off as easily dealt with, further investigation may find that they have been problematic but difficult to articulate, or that it has been difficult to find a suitable person to confide in.

3. Even rather abstract cultural values, such as social integration and cultural inwardness, appear to be related to health. Although the mechanism for such links is unclear these relationships may be important for health planning and policy making. It is therefore important not to discount research findings simply because they do not indicate how to work with individuals. Such findings may be of great importance to public health planners.

4. Cultural inwardness may be a health-promoting attitude which community clinicians can utilize as a resource. Clinicians may therefore build on this by investigating how their interventions can incorporate cultural values and practices. Beyond this, clinicians should resist being seen as a representative of 'modernity' with concomitant bio-technological skills and aligned to moves away from tradition.

5. Some cultural groups, such as the Seventh-Day Adventists, appear to have a healthier lifestyle than other cultural groups. Clinicians must remain open to the possibility of finding healthier ways of living than that prescribed by their own culture or their own profession. Clinicians should make a case for healthier living by referring to outcome data from controlled studies and avoiding evaluative comparisons about what is the 'right' way to live.

6. Different cultural groups experience different diseases to varying extents. This arises through diseases which are genetically determined, acquired, iatrogenic or related to socioeconomic conditions, in addition to those which are influenced by other cultural factors. Acknowledging that some diseases have genetic causes which may be more strongly associated with certain physical features (such as skin colour) than others need not be seen as problematizing culture.

7. Cultures vary in the way in which they understand human body functioning. A balance metaphor appears to be the most common way of viewing the internal working of the body. This metaphor need not be inconsistent with the way in which health professionals work with their clients. Practitioners should try to translate their own thinking into the metaphors used by the cultures they are working with.

8. Explanations for disease varies not only across cultures but with the health professions found within one culture. Many disagreements between health professionals can be understood better if they are seen in, and analysed through, a cultural perspective. Here the challenge is to be able to communicate meaningfully with, and understand, the position of other people.

9. The topic of pain has attracted much cross-cultural research which has led clinicians to develop somewhat stereotypical ideas about how different cultural groups experience pain. Recent research suggests that different cultural groups report similar responses to pain, but that different factors influence these responses. Clinicians should not assume that a lower level of pain complaint or declining the offer of pain killers is associated with a lower level of experienced pain. Patients should be given the choice to cope with their pain in ways consistent with their cultural beliefs, even if these are inconsistent with those of the clinician.

10. Community clinicians must develop a role for themselves where they can negotiate for healthy behaviour between

the models of illness offered by their own profession and the community they seek to serve. Neighbouring communities may have quite different ideas about the cause and necessary preventative action for a particular disease.

11. The hunt for the origins of AIDS is an example of how health professionals and the public alike can be racist when confronted with danger or fear. Clinicians need to confront their own role in sometimes promoting racist attitudes, especially when these become institutionalized as part of the establishment, as was the case with the Nazis in Germany.

12. AIDS is also an example of a disease which has affected some minority cultural groups more than others. We need to be aware that some cultural groups will be more at risk from certain diseases than others, not because of the physical characteristics of their bodies, but because of behavioural patterns which may also be linked to socioeconomic conditions.

# 6

# CULTURE AND TREATMENT

The topic of 'treatment', taking into account the many health professionals who might benefit from this book, is so broad that this discussion needs to be tightly circumscribed. However, it is also going to need to be rather general in order to have some relevance across different professions. We cannot therefore specify how Hungarian counsellors should treat the phobia of a Nigerian client, how Scottish dentists should evacuate the cavities of Pakistani children, or how Malaysian physiotherapists ought to remedy the complaints of Australian athletes! Instead we will consider what is involved in a therapeutic encounter. This will mean trying to develop a way of thinking about and approaching intervention which goes beyond making the patient or client the *object* of treatment. Instead we must acknowledge the patient or client as the *subject* of concern, giving credence to their subjective experience and personal construction of their problems. This sort of analysis of treatment is something which may have great value across the scope of clinical encounters.

## PRACTITIONER–CLIENT COMMUNICATION

The way in which people relate to each other reflects social norms and roles. When is the last time you were a patient? You become a 'patient' when you consult a doctor (or some other clinician), regardless of whether there is something wrong with you, or not. When you leave the doctor's consulting room and go to buy a newspaper in the shop next door, you are no longer a 'patient', regardless of whether you continue to adopt, or have just had validated, a 'sick role'. In most cultures there is a well-worn path to becoming legitimately sick. The gatekeepers along the 'Western' biomedical pathway are conventionally general medical practitioners. GPs decide whether the complaints presented to them are legitimate forms of sickness, or not. If a doctor says that there is nothing wrong with you, while you maintain that you are indeed sick, then you may experience some degree of marginalization. Ridley (1994, p. 88) has described the patient's dilemma thus: 'how to present one's symptoms in a way that does justice to one's feelings, without prejudicing one's status as a responsible person (i.e. without being seen to be "making a fuss").' Clearly a knowledge of social norms and rules is central to being able to present as a convincing patient. It should therefore be of no surprise that communication between practitioners and clients from different cultural backgrounds can be highly problematic and indeed prohibit effective health care.

Before considering some of the complexities of cross-cultural practitioner–client communication, first we review some of the difficulties and limitations of such communication between individuals of the same culture. The vast majority of research on this theme has concerned the communication between medical practitioners and the patients who attend them. It is now well established that patients often fail to act on the advice given to them by a doctor. Often this is because patients do not understand what the doctor is trying to communicate to them, or because they fail to remember what it was they understood the doctor to say during the consultation. Consequently patients fail to comply with the doctor's advice and this may well lessen their chances of recovery, or slow their speed of recovery. Approximately one-third to one-half of patients either fail to take their medicine as prescribed, or fail to follow medical advice. Thus patients' compliance with, or adherence to, the doctor's suggestions continues to be an important area of research. The best informed and most skilful of clinicians is only effective to the extent that he or she can influence the behaviour of their patients in the desired direction (e.g. taking medication, avoiding certain foods, attending specialists, etc.). If the clinicians' communication with patients does not afford them this degree of influence, then the potential benefit of their knowledge will not be felt in practice.

Ridley's review of the importance of the healing relationship highlights the neglected area of the influence of faith in healing. We may talk of faith in the practitioner, and faith in the treatment, or the 'placebo effect'. It is amazing how quickly people (including myself!) recover from a headache after taking a tablet for it. Long before any chemical action can have done its work the headache is out of mind. Of course, trials of new drugs try to take this effect into account by using a control procedure which may involve some people receiving a tablet which, despite being inert, looks and tastes the same as the active drug. More sophisticated trials employ placebos which not only look and taste like the active agent, but also produce some of the unwanted (side) effects of the drug being tested. This sophisticated technology of experimental control has evolved because of the well-accepted notion of the placebo effect: the mere act of engaging in pro-health behaviour (e.g. taking a drug) can improve health. If you believe that you are doing something to make yourself better, then this will, to some extent, make you feel better. The often-quoted phrase, 'we should use the new drugs while they still have the power to heal', nicely encapsulates the role of faith in medicine(s). The placebo effect works not just on patients, but on their clinicians too.

The role of faith in practitioners is no less important than it is in medicines. The actions of a clinician can be seen as having a placebo effect. The doctor who looks at your throat and tells you that it will get better soon, is encouraging you to avoid sick role behaviours and to engage in healthful behaviours.

The doctor's reassurance may make you feel better. Similarly the doctor's involvement in prescribing some treatment may give you greater faith in the treatment. However, without faith in your doctor, treatment or no treatment, you may continue to be ill.

Surely I am not the only clinician to avoid certain treatments until my clients have had a chance to establish some faith in me! For instance, if I am working with a person suffering from agoraphobia, in which I think hyperventilation is influential, I would very rarely ask the person to hyperventilate during our first session. Now I can justify this in all sort of ways, and in truth one of them is to allow the person an opportunity to build trust and confidence in my ability to take care of them during a hyperventilation provocation test. Likewise, I would never use hypnosis with someone during our first session.

There are ways of shortcutting the faith-building process. One is to present yourself as a person in whom others can have faith for particular treatments. A doctor may wear a white coat or a stethoscope, 'advertising' his or her status as a trustworthy person and someone with special knowledge (or powers). Someone who advertises as a specialist in hypnosis may use the technique right away. Such 'advertising' is essentially similar to the placebo which looks like the active agent but may not be. Most practitioners, at least in the clinical specialities, believe that it is the techniques they use, rather than their persona or appearance, which are the active agents. While not disregarding their own behaviour or appearance, they see these as assisting the active agent in the treatment, of which they are but a conduit. However, clinicians may also have faith invested in them by their patients and sometimes this faith may exceed the clinician's ability to deal with the patient's ailment. This presents us with a rather tantalizing notion, that of the 'placebo practitioner' . . . .

What exactly would a placebo practitioner be? It would be somebody who looks like and perhaps acts like a competent practitioner but who doesn't have access to truly therapeutic tools (e.g. effective medicines, techniques or procedures). The theme of placebos and faith is highly relevant to health practices across different cultures. Within one culture the idea of the placebo practitioner is at the root of much professional rivalry. Alternative, or complementary, practitioners are often castigated as presenting themselves as having therapeutic knowledge but in fact being inert. Furthermore, within conventional health services the jibe that some specialists may look good but are not very effective is not unheard of. When we consider practitioners from a different culture the situation becomes even more complex. We may well accept that people from their own culture have some faith in them, but we dismiss the efficacy of their methods. For instance, we may not believe that the amalgam of various herbs presented by an Indian traditional healer has any intrinsic value in alleviating an illness, but we may acknowledge that the way it is prescribed does have a therapeutic effect. Figures 6.1 and 6.2 outline some of these relationships.

Figure 6.1 portrays a matrix of faith in clinicians and their treatments in a monocultural context. In this hypothetical situation there is only one sort of clinician and one sort of treatment. The patient or client either has faith in the treatment or doesn't, and either has faith in the clinician or doesn't. This analysis at the micro-level of the individual indicates that the double placebo condition of faith in both the clinician and the treatment renders the best chance for the recipient of their joint efforts. For instance, I go to my GP, whose professional competence I greatly respect, and she prescribes me a drug, which I understand has been highly effective in treating my sort of problem. In contrast, the scenario in Quadrant 4 might go something like this: I go to a GP whom I have previously found to be rather rude, lacking in sympathy and unable to prescribe effective treatment. He tells me to take a drug which I have taken before and found not only to be ineffective, but also to have unpleasant 'side' effects.

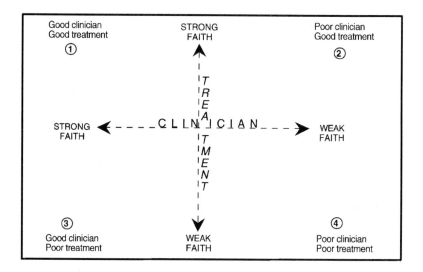

**Figure 6.1:** Faith matrix for clinicians and treatments in a hypothetical monocultural context

Quadrant 2 describes the situation where although one doesn't like the individual doctor, one still believes that the treatment prescribed will be effective. Finally, in Quadrant 3 we have the situation where, although we feel that the doctor is a lovely fella, we also believe that there is no effective medicine for the ailment. In these two latter cases the placebo effects of faith are still present but perhaps modified.

Figure 6.1 makes the assumption that the general therapeutic approach of the clinician (or healer) and the general mode of treatment (or intervention) is acceptable to the client or patient. Thus the patient accepts that their condition should be treated, for example, by a 'Western' medical practitioner (healer) using pharmacological methods (intervention). Clearly this simplistic assumption does not hold even for people of the same cultural background who may differ in their opinions as to the most appropriate sort of person and means of intervention, for a particular problem. The cross-cultural perspective extends this complexity into numerous different understandings about health and illness, how they are caused, who should treat them and in what way.

Figure 6.2 provides a generic matrix for understanding this broader, or macro-level, interaction between faith in the healer and faith in the intervention. At this level Quadrant A represents the situation where the sort of intervention the person is looking for (say, a spell of protection) is the same as the intervention being offered by the healer, and the healer appears to be able to produce an effective intervention of this sort (their spell of protection will indeed afford protection to the recipient). Thus both the mode of intervention and the

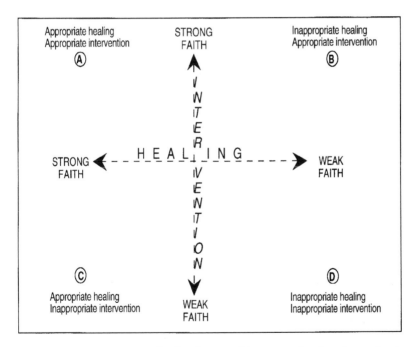

**Figure 6.2:** Faith matrix for healing and intervention in a hypothetical multicultural context

healer to carry out the intervention are seen as appropriate. In Quadrant D neither of these conditions exists.

An example of this might be a Chinese student in Australia going to the college medical practitioner for relief of pain. The student feels that the most appropriate help for his problem would be given by a healer familiar with traditional Chinese ideas of energy imbalances and that the most appropriate treatment would be acupuncture. The Australian doctor, naturally enough, sees the problem from the perspective of his own training and prescribes medication to lessen the patient's experience of pain. Unfortunately he dismisses the student's ideas as unscientific and primitive and is experienced by the student as being rude. The student consequently lacks faith in the healer and the intervention. It is worth reflecting on this for a moment. It has been argued that having faith in both the intervention method and the healer can engage a double placebo effect, such that the patient is helped to get better, partly due to this faith. A lack of faith in both the healer and the method of intervention may not only remove this positive placebo effect, but it may actually produce a negative effect, and may worsen the health of the individual. Such negative consequences may well result from the situation described in Quadrant 4 of Figure 6.1, but it is likely to be even greater when an individual experiences a mismatch between their own philosophy of health and that of a healer they consult. For immigrants or cultural minorities this may enhance feelings of alienation, marginalization and isolation. This undermining of their psychological state may well result in a further deterioration in the condition they are presenting with, or the addition of other problems.

Quadrant B of Figure 6.2 could represent the situation of a general practitioner conducting acupuncture where the patient feels that this is the right sort of intervention, but lacks faith in the GP's knowledge of the technique and ability to carry it out. Such instances may be particularly frustrating for practitioners who attempt to be more eclectic in their practice by also offering 'alternative' therapies. Paradoxically, in the present example, the GP may be ineffective with a Chinese patient who has faith in the technique but lacks faith in the healer, while being effective with an Australian patient, who lacks faith in the technique but has faith in the healer. This latter case is the scenario represented by Quadrant C in Figure 6.2.

The interaction of faith has been examined at the micro-level of individual clinicians and treatment, and at the macro-level of different types of healer and intervention. In reality both of these levels interplay when a person seeks help from a healer and the healer suggests a particular intervention. Figure 6.3 subsumes the previous two figures, representing them on three dimensions. There are 16 different combinations possible through this matrix. For example, A1 represents a match between the sort of healer and sort of intervention a person is seeking and that which is offered, as well as believing in the ability of the individual healer encountered and in the particular treatment recommended.

D3 describes the situation where somebody goes to a healer (for instance a GP) whom they do not see as having the necessary skills to alleviate their problem (for instance, feeling anxious because someone has put a spell on them, or because they have been made unemployed) and also where the sort of intervention (e.g. medication) being offered is not seen as an appropriate method of helping. Nonetheless, they see the clinician as a very nice person who is truly trying to help, but the diazepam prescribed as being of no help. Such complexities may produce confusion and conflict both within the patient and within the clinician, but also *between the two of them*. Their frustration with a mismatch between their two paradigms may spill over to an uneasy relationship between them.

Clearly some of the permutations in Figure 6.3 are more likely than others. Some of them may occur very rarely, if at all. The frequency with which they do occur is open to empirical investigation. If we take seriously the positive influence which

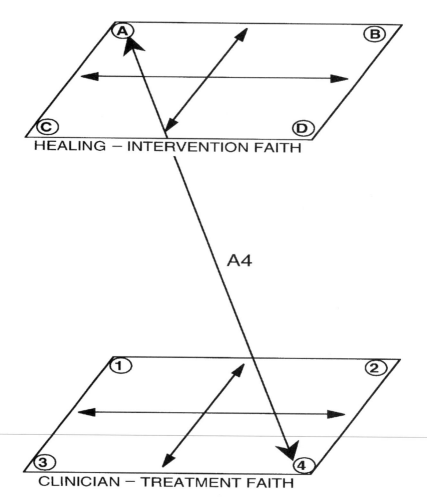

HEALING – INTERVENTION FAITH

A4

CLINICIAN – TREATMENT FAITH

**Figure 6.3:** Faith matrices illustrating a possible interaction between the micro-level of clinicians and treatments, and the macro-level of healers and interventions

belief in a treatment and belief in a healer may have, then it is important to analyse where client–clinician interactions lie within this two-dimensional grid. It is likely that a person's coordinates on this grid have a significant impact on their recovery from an illness or a distressing experience. The grid is intended to emphasize the dual effects which faith in healers and faith in interventions can have on the recovery of a client or patient. It is also intended to help the clinician to think-through where they are in relation to the people they are trying to help. The 'Faith Grid' may be especially useful in understanding the therapeutic process between people from different cultures, or subcultures. We now consider one particular way in which culture influences the interaction between clinicians and clients of the **same** culture.

## Diagnostic disclosure

The idea that 'treatment begins with assessment' is central to many health professions. However, what then becomes of the assessment? A particularly sensitive part of assessment is the decision as to whether the clinician's opinion should be shared with the patient. While such diagnostic disclosure is common in some cultures, there is by no means a universal understanding, either among clinicians or among patients or their families, as to what extent diagnostic information should be disclosed. As expectations about diagnostic disclosure vary across cultures, the practitioner should be aware of how such differences can operate.

Of course within any one culture there will be great variation in the extent to which patients actively seek information about their condition and in the extent to which clinicians feel it is appropriate and/or helpful for the patients to know their condition, especially if they have a poor prognosis. However, psychological research has suggested that certain people do benefit from knowing their prognosis, even if it is poor. It has also been shown that some surgical patients who receive information about their condition, treatment and rehabilitation, prior to being operated on, make a better recovery than those given less information (Anderson, 1987). However, much of this research has been undertaken in North America and no doubt, to some extent, reflects cultural norms such as openness, democracy, individualism and so on. Seen from another point of view, say a Japanese perspective, North American diagnostic disclosure may be experienced as mechanical, direct, blunt, thoughtless and irresponsible. Japanese attitudes towards diagnostic disclosure can be quite different from North American attitudes, and naturally these reflect different aspects of life which are valued in each society. An especially notable difference is in clinician's attitudes towards the disclosure of a diagnosis of mental disorder.

It appears that in Japan there is a particularly strong stigma attached to the diagnostic label of schizophrenia, and that Japanese clinicians often substitute a less stigmatizing diagnosis in their discussions with such patients and their families. It may be argued that, historically, this has its roots in a context of authoritarian clinicians dealing with uneducated patients who were expected to comply with instructions; any serious challenging of an expert's opinion being seen as an arrogant assault on their authority. However, in offering a less severe diagnosis to a person suffering with mental disorder, the clinician may also be seen as assuming a paternalistic and protective role. McDonald-Scott and her colleagues (1992), from the Japanese National Institute of Mental Health, describe this practice as 'benevolent diagnostic deception'. They have investigated this 'deception' by comparing the diagnostic practices of North American and Japanese psychiatrists.

The psychiatrists, all of whom were affiliated with medical schools, were presented with six case vignettes and for each case they indicated if they would tell the patient their diagnosis. The case vignettes represented a variety of clinical conditions. Over 90 per cent of both North American and Japanese psychiatrists said that they would inform patients of a diagnosis of affective or anxiety disorder. However, where the psychiatrist believed the patient to be schizophrenic, only 70 per cent of North American and less than 30 per cent of Japanese psychiatrists would disclose their diagnosis to the patient. In general, Japanese psychiatrists preferred to give a vague alternative diagnosis such as of neurasthenia. This relatively greater reluctance of Japanese psychiatrists to disclose the schizophrenic diagnostic label persisted even in the case where a patient presented with a five-year history of continuous psychopathology and specifically asked if he had schizophrenia or psychosis. This illustrates how powerfully cultural values can influence clinical practice. Clinicians are themselves the vehicles of culture and respond to the broader context in which they are consulted. We might therefore also find that patients' expectations of diagnostic disclosure vary across cultures.

A further aspect of the study by McDonald-Scott *et al.* was that the psychiatrists were asked to indicate whether they would inform the patient's family of the diagnosis. The majority of both Japanese and North American psychiatrists indicated that they would disclose a schizophrenic diagnosis to the patient's family. However, this statistical similarity belies an important cultural difference. North American psychiatrists would disclose the diagnosis to family members only with the patient's permission, while Japanese psychiatrists would do so while neither informing the patient of the diagnosis nor seeking his or her permission to tell family members. Once again this difference may be explained in terms of cultural values. The critical relationship for the North American psychiatrist is between the clinician and the patient, the patient's autonomy being highly valued and the patient's family seen as a distinct, somewhat distant and ethically separate entity. In contrast, for the Japanese psychiatrist the burden of care for the patient is likely to fall on the family. Furthermore, other family members may be seriously jeopardized by a diagnosis of schizophrenia within the family, with its attendant social stigma. Here the psychiatrist has a wider social responsibility which can be fulfilled without informing the patient of his or her condition. Thus what is seen as 'benevolent diagnostic disclosure' in one culture may be classified as malpractice in another. Likewise, adhering to the confidentiality of the clinician–patient relationship in one culture may be regarded as gross social irresponsibility in another.

## Service utilization

Before we proceed with an assumption that communication about health occurs only when a patient gets to the consulting room, let us briefly consider how culture may influence what gets into the clinic. One aspect of this is to consider to what extent available services actually get used. Sue (1994) has stressed the importance of understanding the role of 'shame' and of protecting (saving) 'face' in the underutilization of health services by Asian groups in North America. Related to our previous discussion on diagnostic disclosure, 'Haji' among Japanese, 'Mentz' among Chinese, 'Chaemyun' among Koreans and 'Hiya' among Filipinos are terms used to convey concern over shame or loss of face. The individuals with problems such as juvenile delinquency, AIDS or depression may be seen as bringing disgrace on their whole family. While people from many cultures may be reluctant to publicly engage health services—and by doing so to publicly admit they have problems—Sue argues that this tendency is especially pronounced among Asians. Such cultural differences in services utilization have serious consequences for attempts to provide health across cultures on an equitable basis.

Behaviours associated with shame or stigma are likely to be denied or under-represented to the clinician, perhaps leading to the mistaken conclusion that certain problems are less common in particular cultures. Thus the demand for services may not be equivalent to the need for services. The concept of the 'clinical iceberg', where only a small proportion of clinical problems are ever presented to clinicians, is well accepted. If we assume that all cultural groups have roughly equivalent service needs, this second point would essentially mean that some 'icebergs' are more buoyant than others, and that they are more selectively buoyant. Thus Asians, or any other cultural group, may have service needs which are not met because their culture 'discourages' recognition of particular problems. Even when appropriate services do exist, their uptake may be delayed, or only used as a last resort, with the result that the time-line of a disorder may appear different from one culture to another.

Where the distressed person is not the person who decides to seek professional help, cultural factors may also skew the presentation of problems. For instance, the high achievement orientation of many immigrant Asian families has been noted in North America, Europe, Australia and Africa. Where the admission of a problem may influence a child's opportunities for success, parents can be reluctant to seek appropriate help through formal channels. Thus there are many reasons why the expression and presentation of symptoms to a practitioner may be influenced by the status of a person's problem within their own culture. Likewise the estimation of service needs, as opposed to service demand or service utilization, within any one culture may require great cultural sensitivity on behalf of service providers. Thus cultural variations in help-seeking behaviour need to be taken into account.

As indicated at the beginning of this chapter, 'treatment' must not be thought of only as something which occurs between a clinician and a client or patient. Treatment has to be conceived of as being much broader than this. Following his review of the literature on mental health among Asians, Sue (1994) targets three levels of intervention. At the first level, i.e. individual therapists, he recommends the education and training of therapists around the challenge of how psychotherapeutic issues can be integrated with a client's cultural background. At the next level, i.e. Asian families and communities, he advocates the promotion of positive health messages concerning how stigmatised problems can be successfully treated. For administrators and policy makers, the third level, Sue recommends the recruitment of more Asian therapists, more funding of research on cultural factors which may determine health, and the creation and financing of truly integrated training and treatment programmes.

These points are similar to those made by many others in trying to advance interventions for different cultural groups. One key aspect in such suggestions is the cardinal importance of working through the medium of the client's cultural assumptions. However, cultures change.

> 'Culture' cannot be thought of as a bag of memories and survival techniques which individuals carry about with them and of which they have forgotten to divest themselves. Rather it is a dynamic re-creation by each generation, a complex and shifting set of accommodations, identifications, explicit resistances and reworkings.
>
> (Littlewood, 1992a, p. 8).

All cultures are in a process of change, even those that are replicating their present state. Transition is a part of every 'stable' culture; it is the means through which a social group reproduces a likeness of itself as a social group.

## CULTURAL ASPECTS OF PSYCHOLOGICAL TREATMENTS

Psychotherapies are products of their culture. Many cultures assume that their own culture is the closest interpretation of reality. Most cultures, defining the world in their own way, are understandably self-centred, or ethnocentric, the inhabitants of one culture often seeing the behaviour of members of another culture as being a variation (reinterpretation) of themes within their own culture. In essence, each culture assumes some degree of universalism: that other peoples are like themselves in some important respects. Clearly many cultures also assume that there are some important differences and if these are seen in a negative light then they can be the source of racism. Many 'Western' societies put great value on objectivity and the scientific method. One tenet of the scientific method is that we should study universal laws. In the 'West' there is therefore a (perhaps unconscious) drive to show that different phenomena throughout the world behave according to certain basic universal principles. Thus 'Western' science believes that it should be able to discover these universal laws. If it can do so, then it will be showing that whatever goes on in the world and wherever it happens, these things can be accounted for by rules and principles which reflect the 'Western' way of seeing the world.

There need be nothing sinister in this sort of endeavour. There need be no conspiracy, nor any explicit attempt to colonize the minds of other cultures. Yet there is a real sense in which attempts to apply a psychological treatment developed in one culture to the inhabitants of another culture may be imposing a theory of mind on people who have their own minds and their own theories. Psychologists, or others working through psychological treatments, therefore run the risk of unwittingly becoming missionaries of the mind where they are the agents of a sort of 'Western' psychological colonialism. When psychotherapies developed in the 'West' are practised on members of a cultural group which is relatively disempowered (for instance, immigrants or people in developing countries), then they may deny the validity and dignity of another human being's experience of the world. They may subjugate another person's distress to a foreign language where it cannot be heard, understood or alleviated. This is surely a most damning instance of 'therapeutic' psychology.

A counter-instance of psychology being applied across cultures within this therapeutic domain is where one culture is not necessarily disempowered relative to another, and there is an exchange of ideas between the two. An example of this might be the adoption of Zen Buddhism in some 'Western' psychotherapeutic models, the use of Indian Yoga exercises in 'Western' stress management training or the practise of

Chinese acupuncture in 'Western' pain clinics. These are no lesser examples of one culture influencing another. The millions of people who make up the hundreds of different 'Western' cultures are no less subject to the possibility of hegemony (both from within and outside the 'West') than are those from South American, African or Asian cultures. The important difference is, however, that where a power imbalance exists then there is a danger of one culture's way of seeing the world being (often deliberately) imposed on another.

Check into a hotel in 'down town' Harare, 'grab' a shower, 'flake out' on the bed and 'flick on' the TV. If this is your *modus operandi* then you may not experience the next step: feeling like wallpaper, with CNN coming at you from around the world—that is, the USA world! The 'West' is in your bedroom. It's probably in your TV, your clothes and, before long, your thinking. This is where we are at. Modern technology and power imbalances can colonize minds in peacetime, probably more effectively than they ever could in time of war. Usually in war there is a concerted effort at 'counter-propaganda'. Yet in peacetime where clear dependency relationships exist (again, for instance, between host nationals and immigrants, or between the more and less industrialized countries), the mobilization of cultural forces necessary for resisting such influences may be lacking. Some practitioners who work with culturally disempowered groups are well aware of these problems, yet it is often in those who are most unaware of these problems that the greatest opportunities for change lie. Perhaps you are one of them.

Psychoanalysis is one of the icons of 'Western' psychotherapy. Its originator, Sigmund Freud, was a Jewish German. Many of the early psychoanalysts in Britain were of Jewish origin (having fled the Nazis in the 1930s), yet at that time Britain was also quite anti-Semitic. However, rather than psychoanalysis being developed as a Germanic-Jewish therapy (which might have happened without the Second World War) it was identified with 'science', by postulating that certain intrapsychic processes were common to all people. This particular group of immigrants to Britain was unusual in that they were upper middle class and able to influence the health beliefs of another culture. Their influence was at the significant level of the intellectual British bourgeoisie who were willing to part with their money for this new Germanic-Jewish therapy. The therapy did not explicitly tackle issues of culture but instead focused on the inner life of the individual, safe from the sociopolitical context in which analyst and analysand lived. Yet it is within the middle class, with its white, cerebral, and 'Western' subcultures, that psychoanalysis has largely restricted itself. Indeed, even today popular psychoanalytic folklore has it that to benefit from this treatment you must be smart, rich and white. If this is so then it would clearly be a 'culture-bound' treatment. I do not believe that it is, and indeed Freud's recognition of transference and counter-transference provides a mechanism for exploring all that analyst and analysand bring to the therapeutic encounter. The fact that their 'all' reflects not only intrapsychic processes but also cultural factors, may be an aspect of psychoanalysis which has not been sufficiently developed.

## Modifying psychotherapy across cultures

Many subsequent psychological therapies have followed psychoanalysis in their emphasis on individualism and autonomy. So, for instance, the maximization of the client's potential and the successful negotiation of dependency relationships are keystones in many therapies. One line of research has explored how psychological treatments could be modified in order to take account of their application in 'non-Western' cultures.

Varma (1988) has emphasized the close relationships between culture, personality and psychotherapy, and therefore the importance of adapting 'Western' models of psychotherapy if they are to be used in 'non-Western' contexts. Varma's survey of Indian psychiatrists suggested a number of ways in which this could be done in the Indian context. It was recommended that the therapist should be more active in his or her role, making more directive suggestions and giving reassurance, and putting less emphasis on psychodynamic interpretations. Therapy should be brief, crisis-orientated, supportive and flexible. It should also be eclectic (drawing on a range of techniques from different 'schools') and tuned to the cultural and social conditions, including a recognition of, and blending with, religious beliefs. Finally, it was also suggested that the same level of professional training (as is usual in the 'West') would not be necessary to carry out this function in India.

Ilechukwa (1989), practising psychotherapy in Nigeria, notes a number of points which prohibit the benefits of a 'Western', especially psychodynamic, style of therapy. Perhaps at the most basic level individual therapy ignores the greater sense of collectivism, or group awareness, that prevails in Nigeria in comparison to the USA or Europe. At the level of presentation, Nigerians rarely present with feelings, but with somatic symptoms. The focus is on their physical experience rather than their mental experience. Concerning mode of intervention, the usefulness of the individual approach may be limited; instead, Ilechukwa sees the use of ritualistic therapies, which may help to reintegrate the individual into the group, as being more appropriate. It is also suggested that within the context of psychodynamic therapy many Nigerians find free associating and passivity very threatening. Instead, a more direct approach is advocated, where the therapist tells the client/patient what to do. This, it is argued, falls in with the cultural expectation of being given advice. The practitioner is regarded as *mzee*, a 'powerful stranger'.

Jilek and Jilek-Aall (1984) reviewed several factors which they recommended should be taken into account in psychotherapy with North American Indians. These included the fact that North American Indians generally do not partition 'illness' into the mental and physical dichotomy so often used in

'Western' health care. Furthermore, North American Indians are generally more comfortable with attributing incomprehensible events to supernatural forces, than are 'Westerners' who usually prefer to attribute things beyond their knowledge to knowledge which is waiting—just around the corner—for them to discover. This 'Western' knowledge is, of course, to be unearthed by scientific endeavour. Although 'Westerners' cannot explain it now, they have sufficient faith in their methods to know that, at some point, an explanation in terms of what they currently understand will emerge. Is there not a sense of the supernatural about this? For North American Indians extrapsychic conflicts (that is, social conflicts outside of the self) are seen as more important than interpsychic conflicts (for instance, where parts of the self are in opposition). The focus is again towards the social arena, to social obligations, social status and social living. Here children are seen as universally desired and as an absolute necessity for happiness.

While various authors have emphasized the importance of taking the cultural background of clients into account in therapeutic relationships, others have sought to develop therapy which places culture in the foreground. This is a difficult task and to illustrate this point we now consider the 'culture-centred' approach to psychological therapy.

## Culture-centred intervention

Pedersen and Ivey (1993) have described the 'culture-centred' approach to counselling. Their emphasis is on how the assumptions and values which characterize a particular culture shape and direct the behaviour of individuals within that culture. This they have contrasted with several other approaches to counselling. For instance, a person-centred approach assumes that the individuals are autonomous within their culture and that they have the power to act and think independently of their cultural context. A problem-centred approach sets its sights on solving externalized problems, often neglecting to appreciate the social and cultural function which a 'problem' may be serving for the owner of that problem. Behaviour-centred approaches attempt to manipulate behaviour without consideration for its cognitive or cultural representation. Situation-centred approaches may focus on the context of behaviour (including its cultural context) without taking into account the individual's own interpretation of the situation.

Pedersen and Ivey have attempted to develop a way of acquiring counselling skills that will make counsellors effective across many different cultures. Thus, rather than identifying the requisite skills to work in a particular culture, they attempted to identify skills to work with all cultures. An initial stage of their training programme is to release the practitioners from their own 'cultural encapsulation'. This term, originally used by Wrenn (1962), refers to the practitioners' inclination to use stereotypes of the world in order to make it more manageable and to assume that their own (culture's) aspirations for an individual are also those of their client. The first stage of Pedersen and Ivey's training programme therefore concentrates on making practitioners aware of their own cultural assumptions. The second stage presents a conceptual framework, called the 'Cultural Grid', for distinguishing between personal and cultural aspects of interpersonal and intrapersonal relationships. This grid allows one to consider the variables which influence the values, expectations and behaviours of individuals.

The third stage of the model uses the concept of four 'synthetic cultures'. These synthetic cultures are based on Hofstede's (1980) four dimensions of culture (previously described in Chapter 2). The cultures, described as alpha, beta, gamma and delta, refer to Hofstede's dimensions of small to large power/distance, collectivism–individualism, femininity–masculinity and strong to weak uncertainty avoidance. Practitioners are taught appropriate counselling skills for clients from each of these cultures. The practical value of this approach is that it illustrates how, for instance, different questioning or reflecting skills may be required for individuals from 'alpha' and 'gamma' cultures. Theirs is an interesting and mechanically intricate attempt to provide practitioners with a means of thinking through different cultures. Although Pedersen and Ivey argue for the various advantages of this approach, it is quite problematic.

The four dimensions described by Hofstede were derived from research initiated over 20 years ago, in an industrial not a therapeutic context, with one multinational company and on a data set designed for a different purpose. This is not to detract from the usefulness of Hofstede's analyses, but rather, to recognize their limitations. Can, for instance, 200 employees of IBM in Finland really be taken to be a representative sample of the values of Finnish people? Is it possible to generalize from the views of people 20 years ago to the views of people from the same geographic areas today? In addition to these points there has for some time been concern with Hofstede's interpretation of some of the dimensions, especially the masculine–feminine dimension. This dimension, in particular, would have great significance in the therapeutic domain.

However, the major problem with the synthetic cultures approach is that the cultures are synthetic. They do not exist. They are caricatures, stereotypes based on psychological research which was conducted for a quite different purpose. In attempting to use abstractions for training there is a danger that counsellors will be skilled only in an abstract sense and not in the real sense of working with people from real-world cultures. Here the counsellors may struggle to place the individual, or his or her culture, somewhere along the abstract dimensions which they have been trained to deal with. In doing so they may be distracted from the particular meaning of the presenting problem, for the particular person they are working with. The limitations of Hofstede's empirical dimensions for counselling work with individuals have also been noted elsewhere (e.g. Lago & Thompson, 1996).

In any analysis of culture we must always remain aware that culture works through individual people. Yet culture also provides the social medium through which individuals work through life. Individuals and their culture(s) reciprocally influence each other. Even in the case of individuals who completely reject their cultural heritage, or who feel themselves to be between various cultural heritages, their attitudes can still be described relative to certain cultural values. We therefore return to an issue discussed in Chapter 1, that is, the importance of keeping the individual foreground and the cultural background in perspective, for every person. Since both individuals and cultures are in a process of continual change, this seems a tall order indeed. I now set out an alternative attempt at unravelling this matrix, one that recognizes that our worlds do not necessarily fit neatly into other people's categories, that we may not ourselves be aware of all the cultural and idiosyncratic assumptions which propel us, and one which uses as its primary data the immediacy of personal experience.

## Analysing critical incidents as a therapeutic technique

We wish to find out what individuals consider important in their lives. If we can unravel the goals and rules by which people live their lives then we can get closer to understanding what will make them happy and sad, hopeful and pessimistic, angry and timid. Personality theory, and psychology in general, has attempted to come up with universally applicable explanations of why people are as they are. The search continues for grand theories that might explain the behaviour not just of one individual but of millions of people. In the technique to be described here the focus is idiographic and qualitative. We are concerned with how individuals experience life in their own terms. We are not particularly concerned to compare this experience to that of others, to say whether it is more or less, better or worse, happier or sadder. The therapeutic use of critical incidents, which I am suggesting here, has its roots in occupational (or industrial) psychology and so to put it into some kind of context let us briefly consider this.

The technique of critical incidents analysis was first described by Flanagan (1954) for use in the context of industrial psychology. Here a key question was: 'What sort of skills are necessary to carry out a particular work role?' However, rather than the 'experts' in industrial psychology being asked this question, the question was directed at the 'on-the-job experts', those actually doing the job being studied. Now simply asking somebody what skills are necessary for them to do their job is a deceptively easy question. In fact we may often not know exactly what skills we use, perhaps because we have become over-familiar with our work role. Flanagan therefore asked the same question in a different way. First of all he asked workers to define the objectives of their job, not as stated by their boss or in the company manual, but in their own terms. Second, they were asked to describe incidents that were critical to their achieving the objectives which they had described. The incidents could be critical in the positive sense of helping them to achieve their objectives, or negative in the sense of prohibiting them from achieving their objectives. Having thus identified a balance of positive and negative critical incidents, the workers were asked to reflect on the skills they used (or failed to use) during these incidents that were relevant to achieving their work objectives. In this way a catalogue of skills relevant to the job was built up.

Recently this approach has been used to identify job skills, not in the context of industry, but for people working with traumatized refugees. We will therefore review some examples from my own research to illustrate the critical incident technique in a domain more clearly relevant to health and welfare work across cultures (Kanyangale & MacLachlan, 1995). During the height of the Mozambican war over one million Mozambican refugees poured into neighbouring Malawi. Many of these people had been traumatized through their war experiences. Relief work has usually (and understandably) targeted the immediate physical health needs of refugees. However, a sole focus on physical health neglects the fact that such efforts may be inhibited in their effectiveness by the mental state of traumatized refugees. Their trauma is, of itself, deserving of therapeutic intervention. In collaboration with the Finnish Refugee Council we investigated the job experiences of 15 counsellors who were themselves also refugees. Table 6.1 shows the objectives identified by those counsellors who were working with traumatized children.

The following is an example of a critical incident given by a counsellor who was working with a young boy:

**Table 6.1:** Objectives of counsellers of Mozambican refugee children

| Statement of objective | Frequency |
| --- | --- |
| (1) To play a variety of games with refugee children so that they can forget their war experience | 5 |
| (2) To encourage group sharing of personal war experiences | 3 |
| (3) To change the depressive feelings and thoughts of refugee children affected by war by inducing their participation in activities | 3 |
| (4) To give advice to refugee children through telling them meaningful stories | 3 |
| (5) To involve refugee children, without their parents, in singing, dancing, and other cultural activities | 2 |
| (6) To create a sense of security | 1 |

Reproduced from Kanyangale and MacLachlan (1995) with permission.

It was time to play football and a certain boy could not play with the others. Every time I tried to make this boy participate, he would complain of pain from a tiny wound on his left leg. On this day I chatted with the boy for a long time behind a fence, and learnt that the child's father was killed in Mozambique. I was also told that peers mock and segregate the boy saying that he is a fool. He stays with his mother and has no father. I also gathered that peers refuse to play with him. I felt sorry and assured the child that he was free to play without being mocked, like any other child in the programme. Currently, the boy leads others in singing and dancing and he is good at riddles. The boy consults me for advice whenever he is provoked.

The counselling skills identified from this incident included the ability to create an environment of security/trust (from giving the child an opportunity to play without the fear of disapproval), the ability to probe (from having investigated the boy's home life and uncovered the fear of disapproval), the ability to communicate a sense of being understood and cared for (from comforting the boy, showing interest and giving reassurance). In addition to these attributes identified by the counsellor himself, we also noted the counsellor's awareness of defence mechanisms (from the counsellor's recognition of the boy's projection of his fears onto the pain from the tiny wound) as an important attribute. The attributes identified from incidents such as these may then be synthesized into related themes.

Table 6.2 shows the complete list of skills identified in this way from 15 refugee counsellors. As can be seen, the technique of critical incident analysis provides rich qualitative information based on the acknowledgement of expertise which lives within the individual who is actually doing the job. This technique may therefore have the potential of uncovering some of the clinical skills, which particularly effective cross-cultural practitioners use, as well as highlighting the circumstances which many of us find particularly difficult to deal with. Because the technique is so practically focused in

**Table 6.2:** Job-related attributes identified by refugee counsellors

| | Frequencies | | |
|---|---|---|---|
| Attributes | +ive | –ive | Total |
| *Interview process* | | | |
| Create a sense of security and trust | 4 | 6 | 10 |
| Communicate a sense of being understood and cared for | 1 | 8 | 9 |
| Sympathy | 4 | 5 | 9 |
| Tolerance | 4 | 7 | 11 |
| Patience | 3 | 4 | 7 |
| Sensitivity to individual's needs | 1 | 2 | 3 |
| Non-judgemental | 1 | 3 | 4 |
| Prompt verbal communication | 7 | 3 | 10 |
| Facilitate open discussion | 3 | 3 | 6 |
| Probing | 4 | 5 | 9 |
| *Analytical skills* | | | |
| Interpret emotional reactions to be reasonable and normal | 5 | 3 | 8 |
| Challenge assumptions | 2 | 1 | 3 |
| Awareness of defence mechanisms* | 2 | 3 | 5 |
| Identify reinforcers of maladaptive behaviour | 4 | 5 | 9 |
| Sensitivity to emotional readiness to confront painful experiences* | 1 | 3 | 4 |
| Observe abnormal behavioural patterns | 7 | 6 | 11 |
| Awareness of step-by-step progression towards goal achievement* | 1 | 2 | 3 |
| Awareness of non-verbal behaviour | 1 | 1 | 2 |
| *Self in relation to others* | | | |
| Perception of self and others* | 3 | 1 | 4 |
| Being flexible in problem solving | 1 | 4 | 5 |
| Awareness of the influence of power relationships on communication* | 1 | 1 | 2 |
| Sensitivity to the communicative function of physical contact* | 3 | 4 | 7 |

\* Identified by interviewer.
Reproduced from Kanyangale and MacLachlan (1995) with permission.

terms of applied clinical skills, and because it acknowledges and utilizes the skills of people actually doing clinical work, it could act as an important adjunct to training in therapeutic skills. However, the technique may also be able to make a more direct contribution to the clinician's approach to treatment across cultures.

Because the critical incident technique describes authentic or real scenarios its value has been recognized for training in cross-cultural awareness. Brislin *et al.*'s (1986) cultural assimilator presents a series of critical incidents drawn from a range of different cultural settings. The trainee must choose the most culturally appropriate response from several alternative possibilities. Explanations are provided for each choice. By realizing the rationale for their correct responses as well as the reasons for their errors, trainees are helped to assimilate a degree of sensitivity to issues of culture, especially communication across cultures. In addition to cross-cultural training, critical incidents have also been used to enhance clinical skills in various settings.

The original technique of critical incidents analysis sought to identify appropriate skills, or behaviours, from people 'on the job'. Critical incidents were defined as those incidents which specifically related to a person's job objectives. As such the objectives of the job defined the sort of incidents to be discussed, whether they were examples of the use of appropriate skills or of skills lacking.

In living, we are already doing a job. Every day we experience incidents which are critical to our mental and physical well-being. We find ourselves pleased with the outcome of some important events and disappointed with the outcome of others. Can we not, therefore, determine what our objectives must be? If we can determine a person's objectives for living, then we are some way towards understanding how culture, family relationships, personal aspirations and so on interact within any one of us. Thus, by examining what a person's critical incidents are we can work backwards to unearthing their objectives. Sometimes we will do things for reasons which are perfectly clear to us, yet at other times our own behaviour can be a bit of a mystery. Conflicts between cultural identities for members of immigrant groups may be traced, for example, to conflicts in their objectives of living, where one objective is to retain traditional values, while another objective is to be accepted into the host society. These and other factors form important elements in the following case study, which explicates the technique I have described as 'critical therapy'.

---

*Case Study: A Cross-Cultural Example of Critical Therapy*

*Shagufta is a 16-year-old girl whose family came to England from Pakistan three years after she was born. The family has returned to Pakistan twice since, on holidays, where Shagufta has enjoyed meeting with her extended family and taking part in family celebrations. In England, she is an excellent pupil at the local comprehensive school and is popular both with other Asian girls and among the (majority) white English pupils. For the past six months Shagufta has been caught in a 'Bulimic cycle' where she binges on sweet foods, vomits what she has eaten, feels great guilt over having done this and then sometime later binges, vomits and feels guilty again. Shagufta's mother had recently read an article called 'Eating disorders: the modern Western plague'. After discovering her in the middle of vomiting one night and being suspicious of her secretly eating, Shagufta's mother brought her to their general practitioner who referred her to a clinical psychologist for treatment of bulimia nervosa. She has now seen the psychologist twice.*

*Shagufta has continued her bingeing behaviour. Last night at 2.00 a.m. after having binged on biscuits and bread for two hours she was making herself sick, vomiting into the toilet bowl, when she heard somebody coming along the corridor. She speedily cleaned up the vomit around the bowl and flushed the toilet. Her mother knocked on the door and Shagufta came out of the toilet reassuring her mother* that everything was alright and that she had not been vomiting. While in the toilet her mother discovered a patch of vomit which Shagufta has missed. She went to Shagufta's bedroom and there ensued a huge argument. Shagufta describes the incident as a clearly negative incident, identifying the following important aspects:

'I had an argument with my mother.'
'I lied to my mother.'
'I gave in to a desire to binge.'
'I felt so guilty and lonely before the binge.'
'My mother said that she had never heard of anything like this before in Pakistan and that I am shaming my family'
'My mother said I was acting like a silly little English girl.'

To understand how these critical aspects of the incident are related to Shagufta's broader objectives we must ask 'Why are they important?' Sometimes the relevant objective will be quite transparent. For instance, the first two points, in this case, related to a belief that Shagufta should respect her mother. The third point concerns the belief that one should use self-control, behave with some propriety and not over-indulge oneself. The fifth point, concerning how this had never happened to anyone else in the family, was about the expectation that Shagufta should make her parents proud, especially as she showed such promise at school. Shagufta was not sure why the final point should be so annoying to her, but she felt that it was important. Nor could she identify it with any major objective in her life.

In an attempt to clarify this the technique of laddering was used:

QUESTION: What would it mean if you were acting like a silly little English girl?
SHAGUFTA: It would mean that I was being foolish in an English way.
QUESTION: What does it mean to be foolish in an English way?
SHAGUFTA: It means I am not behaving as I should?
QUESTION: How should you behave?
SHAGUFTA: I should try to be sensible . . . I should not try to be English!

QUESTION:    *What does it mean if you should be sensible and not*
             *English?*
SHAGUFTA:    *It means I should be Pakistani.*
QUESTION:    *Is this one of your objectives in life?*
SHAGUFTA:    *I really don't know . . . but it's one of my mother's*
             *objectives for me.*

*Thus the fifth and sixth points identified by Shagufta relate to her*
*ambivalence about an objective which she feels her mother expects of*
*her. Incidentally, the same scenario can also be used to find some-*
*thing positive: the problem was discussed, Shagufta is not being*
*secretive at present and so on. Clearly no two people will interpret*
*an incident in the same way. The practitioner must be guided*
*through the interpretation by their client. The practitioner's skill is*
*in providing a framework to identify objectives and, where necess-*
*ary, asking appropriate questions to clarify them.*

---

The critical incident to be analysed in the form described in
the preceding case study need not be one of emotional out-
burst, it could be a stomach pain, a worry or any incident
which makes the person feel uncomfortable. The strength of
the critical incident process becomes apparent in its reflec-
tivity. That is, identifying the objectives relating to the incident may not simply give the practitioner a better idea of the
cultural context and personal values of their clients, it may
also allow the clients to reflect on the meaning of their problems. In short, it may be therapeutic in itself. However, at the
very least, in the cross-cultural context, it should clarify the
beliefs, values and expectations which clients have and how
these relate to particular problem areas in their lives.
However, no therapeutic technique can be effective if it fails
to take account of the much broader social and cultural context in which therapy is being sought and offered. The work
of the Nafsiyat Centre has been distinctive in confronting and
integrating this perspective in its clinical work.

## INTERCULTURAL THERAPY

Nafsiyat Intercultural Therapy Centre was established in London in 1983 to provide a specialist psychotherapy service to minority cultural groups. The centre provides a clinical service, training courses for health personnel, consultation to clinicians in related fields, and undertakes research into the efficacy of therapy. Kareem, the founder and clinical director of Nafsiyat, describes the objective of intercultural therapy as being '. . . to create a form of therapeutic relationship between the therapist and patient where both can explore each other's transference and assumptions. This process attempts to dilute the power relationship that inevitably exists between the "help giver" and the "help receiver".' (Kareem, 1992, p. 16). We will shortly unpack this description. Before doing so, it is important to appreciate that Kareem's approach to therapy, unlike many contemporary alternatives, acknowledges that individuals' distress results not necessarily from within themselves but from much broader economic and sociopolitical influences which colour the context in which they experience the world. Therapy, therefore, becomes a means for understanding the various factors—social, political, economic, psychological, cultural—which may contribute to the creation of distress experienced by members of cultural minorities. Thus, prejudice, racism, sexism, poverty, social disadvantage and the internalization of these experiences are confronted as tools of social injustice which may fully account for the distress with which a person presents. Hopefully intercultural therapy also becomes an occasion for empowerment and self-affirmation of minority cultural groups and individuals.

Intercultural therapy is based on a psychodynamic model. We have already noted that any therapy is a product of certain cultural assumptions. However, it has also been argued that this need not prohibit the application of certain therapeutic techniques outside their culture of origin. One psychodynamic therapeutic technique which may have wide relevance is the interpretation of transference and counter-transference. This is an important element of intercultural therapy. Transference refers to the idea that in any encounter between two people there is also an encounter between two histories. These histories may be consciously or unconsciously presented.

A simple example would be where a client in therapy was behaving towards the therapist, and other authority figures, as though they were his father. The client is transferring the feelings he has about his father into his relationship with his therapist. In turn his therapist also has a personal history. Again he may be consciously aware of certain ways in which his past experiences influence his current relationships but he may also be unaware of other ways in which his past experiences are influencing the way he relates to his client. The therapist too may transfer his feelings, perhaps about his son, onto the client who relates to him in a paternal role. This describes the counter-transference. In this example the therapeutic encounter is explicitly between the therapist and his client, yet implicitly it may be between the client's father and the therapist's son. Psychotherapists therefore may 'work through' and make interpretations about 'the transference'.

Personal histories are not just about what has happened to an individual. They are also about the way in which an individual has come to understand the world and his or her place in it. Personal histories reflect culture, heritage and social history. Building on our simplified example, if the client is black and his father worked on a colonial run British tobacco farm in Africa, and the therapist is white and his father was in the British colonial service, then what histories do they each bring to this encounter? How do their histories interplay? What assumptions does each make about the other? And so on. It would be very surprising if an encounter between a 'help-seeking' member of a disempowered cultural minority and a 'help-giving' member of the white, middle-class intellectual élite did not have some resonance (perhaps literal but more usually symbolic) with their cultural histories. How such factors interact with other aspects of their transference and how these should be worked through is beyond the focus of this book. But it is to this hinterland of culture and health that intercultural therapy addresses itself.

Littlewood (1992a), another proponent of intercultural therapy, emphasizes that there can be no 10-point prescription for the clinician working across cultures. He also states that intercultural therapy should not be allowed to become a specialized psychotherapy targeted only at one culturally defined section of a society. Instead, intercultural therapy is simply therapy which acknowledges and confronts the broader sociocultural context in which we all operate, whether as members of a powerful majority or of a repressed minority. In this sense we are all potentially 'part of the solution' because we are all an element in the matrix of the problem. For the therapist of white European descent Littlewood (1992b, p. 41) powerfully encapsulates the dilemma thus: 'The obvious "liberal" approach is one which simply seeks to offer the European therapeutic model to others on the basis that this is the best we have and that common justice invites us to extend its application. Unless the very problem for which we extend it is ourselves?' For example, if black people present with distress (psychological or physical problems) which result from their negative experience of white dominance over blacks, then offering them 'white' therapies is problematic. It may be seen as denying the legitimate expression of oppression, by transforming its consequences (distress) into a form of pathology treatable by 'white' medicine. In short, it adds insult (of superior white intervention) to the injury (of oppression of black people). This is without doubt an extreme sociopolitical interpretation, but not one without value. It is unfortunate because it pits one culture against another, which is neither necessary nor desirable. An interesting recent approach to therapy for relatively disempowered groups has been to embellish the value of their cultural perspective. Reclaiming one's culture may be incorporated as a key element in reclaiming a healthy self-identity. Let us examine how this can work in settings as diverse as Canada, Australia and Scotland.

## CULTURE AS TREATMENT

Alcoholism and drug abuse are a major problem among many indigenous minorities, in both rural and urban settings. Brady (1995), of the Australian Institute of Aboriginal and Torres Strait Islander Studies, has reviewed the high incidence of alcoholism among First Nations North Americans (American and Canadian 'Indians') and Australian Aborigines, and the recent emphasis on the use of 'culture' as a mode of treatment by these groups. These treatment programmes, which attempt to reassert a positive native identity through the practice of traditional customs and the valuing of traditional beliefs, expound the philosophy that *culture is treatment*.

Why has 'culture' become 'treatment'? A good part of the reason for this probably lies in the contemporary indigenous understanding of the cause of drug and alcohol abuse, which attributes these to social deprivation and the erosion of cultural integrity (acculturation) through colonization. The individual alcoholic is seen as a social expression of the experience of cultural repression. Reconnecting individual aborigines with their cultural heritage not only provides a medium for intervention, but also regenerates traditional values which are increasingly being portrayed as counter drug abuse. The Nechi Institute in Alberta is one of the leading indigenous drug abuse treatment centres in Canada. The treatment policy of the centre incorporates various indigenous practices with a disease-based model and an adaptation of the 12 steps used by Alcoholics Anonymous. One of the traditional cultural elements which may form part of the Nechi treatment programme is the sweat lodge. The use of sweat lodges is the most common feature of native alcohol treatment programmes in North America.

The sweat lodge is a sort of ritualized sauna which takes place in a small rounded structure made by placing blankets or canvas over a frame of willow saplings. Inside, a central pit of hot stones is splashed with water in order to produce steam. Participants, usually wearing shorts, sit around the stones in total darkness for several sessions of up to 30 minutes each. Various ritual practices may take place within the sweat lodge and tobacco may be used. While sweat lodges are traditionally used by many indigenous North American groups, it is not common to all of them and the actual purpose of the sweat lodge and its associated rituals may differ from one region to another. Nonetheless it is not attributed to any one tribal or linguistic group and has in recent times been seen as a central part of a broadly based First Nations resurgence. The sweat, through the powerful physical and mental experiences it produces, therefore allows an individual to embrace a sense of cultural reawakening.

Brady suggests four ways in which sweats, while being used as a treatment for alcoholism, are also an important mechanism for the revival and development of a positive cultural identity. First, the sweat is a symbol of Indianness. For those who have lost touch with many aspects of their traditional culture (for example, language or religion) the sweat offers an instant and dramatic way of immersing oneself in Indianness. The second suggestion, relating specifically to alcoholism, is that the 'overwhelming physical sensation of undergoing a sweat is of detoxification and cleansing' (Brady, 1995, p. 1492). It therefore is consonant with the idea of physical, psychological and spiritual purification—a fresh start. Third, the drama of the occasion and the fortitude required to proceed with it, provides a clear rite of passage and demarcation of an individual's commitment to a new way. The final suggestion refers to the sweat leaders. In the treatment programmes these individuals are often ex-drinkers who now serve as positive role models. The sweat helps them to maintain their own sobriety.

While research on the effectiveness of programmes which incorporate traditional elements, such as sweat lodges, is still ongoing, it is their cultural aspects which are of particular interest to us here. The sweat lodge is an intervention both for the individual and for the community. It signifies an alternative to modern Indian life, one which empowers traditional aspects of culture. It endows historical culture with goodness, with wellness and with value.

## Australian aboriginal treatment of alcoholism

A particularly intriguing aspect of the resurgence in First Nations traditional healing methods for alcohol addiction is their adoption by another indigenous group who are geographically distant and culturally distinct, the Aboriginal peoples of Australia. They also are a people who have suffered dispossession of their land, historically poor race relations and woefully inadequate access to health services. Brady describes how a central part of some recent alcohol addiction programmes among Aboriginal peoples has stressed the spiritual relationship with the land. Regaining a meaningful relationship with 'Mother Earth', with the 'Aboriginal Mother', is seen as an important pathway out of alcoholism. Many Aboriginal religious practices and beliefs are linked to features of the landscape, created by their ancestors during the 'Dreaming'. Once again, *'culture'* is being presented *as treatment.*

Addictions are, however, seen as a 'non-traditional' problem among Australian Aborigines and therefore to lie beyond the knowledge of Aboriginal traditional healers. This is one major drawback in seeing 'culture' historically, as traditions and customs from the past. In Aboriginal traditional healing there is no tradition of the group as a therapeutic medium; instead, a healer and client meet on a one-to-one basis in relative privacy. Based on certain commonalities in their historical experiences and their contemporary marginalization, Australian Aborigines have recently innovatively incorporated First Nations North American customs into their treatment programmes for alcoholism. Canadian Indian consultants have been employed to advise on and take part in the development of treatment programmes in Australia. There have been numerous exchanges between the aboriginal peoples of North America and Australia, concerned with incorporating traditional methods into the treatment of addictions. In some centres, North American traditions never previously seen in Australia have been incorporated into treatment programmes. This includes the Medicine Wheel (as a symbol of wholeness and strength), beginning each day by the burning of sweet grasses (as a ceremony of prayer and welcome) and the institution of ritual morning hugs and handshakes. Indeed, according to Brady, a Canadian Indian visiting Western Australia was recently asked to build a sweat lodge.

While we may well have concerns (also expressed by some Australian Aborigines) about the appropriateness of grafting traditional First Nations customs onto contemporary Australian Aboriginal treatments for addiction, Brady makes the much more positive observation that a major synthesis between these two healing traditions is now taking place. Aboriginal treatments for addiction also adhere to the 12 steps (disease model) of Alcoholics Anonymous and incorporate methods for getting people back 'in touch' with 'Mother Earth'. However, it is also recognized that certain aspects of Aboriginal culture, such as a reluctance to confront (interfere with) people who are having personal problems, deriding ('pulling down') those who seek to escape from a (drinking) group norm, perhaps to 'better' themselves in some way, or not using groups as a medium of help, should not be seen as immutable customs.

This Australian situation provokes important questions about health and cultural healing: 'Are the First Nations of North America partially proselytizing Aboriginal Australians?', 'Is the exchange little more than a form of psychological colonialism?' or 'Does this synthesis reflect a recognition of the function of "culture" as a medium for self-affirmation?', 'Is there anything wrong with benefiting from the customs of another culture?'. And, perhaps finally, 'Why is it so important to retain our own cultural heritage if any one will do?' In an attempt to address some of these issues we will briefly consider a long-itudinal study of a four-year long Tibetan Buddhist retreat conducted in Dumfriesshire, Scotland, from 1989 to 1993. This retreat may be seen as another example of 'culture as treatment'.

## The Samye-Ling Retreat: an alternative culture

Buddhism is a religious way of life which is based on the 'awakening' of Siddharta Guatama, later known as Buddha. He was a rich and pampered prince who, lacking fulfilment, decided to turn his back on his privileges and to become home-less. He achieved enlightenment through meditation. Although the contemporary practise of Buddhism varies according to different interpretations, some concepts may be identified as central. The law of *Karma*, or cause and effect, ties people to a cycle powered by the results of their good and evil acts. Through *reincarnation* one must live with the consequence of previous lives. The *Four Noble Truths* of Buddhism describe how suffering is the effect of past karma; how misplaced values, particularly those of material wealth, are self-limiting; how suffering can be overcome and that there is a path to achieve this. This path, known as the *Noble Eightfold Path*, iden-tifies 'right' knowledge, attitude, speech, action, occupation, effort, mindfulness and composure as its basic elements. By following this path the goal of *Nirvana*, a transformed mode of human consciousness, may be reached. Tibetan Buddhism is one particular interpretation of these ideas.

Buddhist ideas have recently become popular in Europe and North America where they represent not only a culturally foreign religion, but also a way of life, a way of being, which is quite foreign too. Various reasons may account for this popularity. Buddhism may be seen as more tolerant than, for instance, Christianity; the order of natural justice—reaping what you sow—may also be appealing, and the high moral standards of Buddhism are certainly praiseworthy.

The Kagya Samye-Ling Tibetan Centre in Scotland was the site for a four-year retreat undertaken by 46 people from all over the world, including each of the five continents. Artists, journalists, engineers, teachers, lawyers, receptionists, nurses, the unemployed and a prisoner on parole were among them. This was the largest Tibetan Buddhist retreat ever undertaken outside of Tibet. As we have described (McAuliffe & MacLachlan, 1994), the retreat involved a number of discrete stages. The first year was dominated by prayers (incorporating chanting and visualization) to remove obstacles to the retreat, to promote long life, 'purify negativity', and develop generosity and a devotion to 'the enlightened beings'. In order to assist the transition from the busy world to the relative tranquillity of retreat, the first year also involved vigorous physical exercise to use up energy and settle the mind. The second year of retreat involved 'shrine (samatta) meditation'. Using techniques such as focusing on breathing helped to 'still the mind' and to prepare the retreater for a six-month period of 'intensive practice', again requiring much chanting and visualization. This period also required retreaters to minimize their activities in order that the mind would have as few distractions as possible. To this end, talking and writing were prohibited for the six months. In the third year of the retreat there was much less chanting, and physical exercise was introduced for one hour each day until the end of the retreat. The third year continued with the more complex prayer and meditative practices used during the 'intensive period', these being seen as the heart of the retreat. In the fourth year simpler practices were used (with less chanting) to help the retreater 'wind down'.

Certain aspects of the retreat no doubt seem quite foreign. For instance, the fact that the retreaters were housed only with members of their own sex and essentially stayed within their retreat houses for the whole four years, suggests the uniqueness of this form of voluntary 'withdrawal'; even more, given that some of the retreaters were married with children and that, in some cases, both partners went into retreat. Also, for a six-month period retreaters abstained from washing. Such 'bizarre' aspects of the retreat's culture surprise or even shock some people. Yet within the ethos of the retreat they make perfect sense. Are there really any cultures in which people knowingly engage in senseless activity? Yet from outside a culture we may not be able to make sense of certain activities. Perhaps the most significant question is: 'Was the retreat's culture of benefit to its participants?'

Participation in our research was voluntary, and although the majority of subjects initially agreed to take part, by the end of the four years only nine people had completed all of our yearly assessments. Many were concerned that our activities might be a distraction from the ethos of the retreat, particularly during the 'intensive period'. We used a range of different quantitative and qualitative techniques to investigate retreaters' experiences. Over the first six months of the retreat (based on data from 29 retreaters) we reported a significant decrease in their sleep disturbance and in their ratings of the severity of personal problems. Despite the substantial transition in their daily lives—which we had expected would be quite stressful—we did not find any significant increase in their reporting of perceived stress or psychological disorder. Three and a half years later there were further significant reductions in the reported severity of personal problems and no increase in perceived stress or psychological disorder, both of which, on average, fell well within the 'normal' range.

Despite this lack of stress 'symptoms' many retreaters did initially describe difficulties with adapting to the retreat. Following this, many indicated a process of becoming increasingly aware of their own limitations, subsequently growing in self-confidence, and then being anxious about the finishing of the retreat. This process of deconstruction and then reconstruction has similarities to some forms of psychotherapy. Wray (1986) has described Buddhism as 'the cultivation of increasingly

ethical conduct, of a concentrated, tranquil but vibrantly ener-
getic and joyful state of mind, and of the subsequent Transcen-
dental Wisdom and compassion arising like a flower on a
healthy plant' (p. 165). Clearly Buddhism offers a unique
perspective on life and how to confront life's problems. In the
case of the Samye-Ling retreat, people from all over the world
were immersed in the culture of Tibetan Buddhism. To the vast
majority of retreaters this culture was very different from the
one in which they were reared and socialized. Indeed, for
some, this may have been the very attraction of Tibetan Buddhism. Inasmuch as the retreat and the religion are seen as a
means to improving people's state of mind and body, then it
too can be seen to be a case of 'culture as treatment'.

# CONCLUSION

Emerging from studies of 'culture as treatment' is the idea
that the attributes of a culture—a context, language, rituals,
symbols, etc.—can offer people a vehicle for confronting their
problems. 'Culture as treatment' may offer a means of countering a sense of cultural anomie, that is, in countering the
aimlessness which a person may experience through the rejection of the norms of his or her original cultural group. In such
cases, 'culture as treatment' offers the individual another 'system of living'.

Treatments are ritualized in different ways in different cultures. Whether we experience healing through sweat lodges,
Mother Earth, psychoanalysis or keyhole surgery may not
matter, but what does matter is that the healing is presented
in a context which gives our experiences meaning. A strong
belief in any particular meaning, be it biomedical science or
spirit possession, is likely to heighten our faith in its
treatments and practitioners. A pluralistic belief in different
modes of intervention may allow us more ways of getting
better. However, it is not simply a matter of adopting a *laissez-
faire* attitude of 'whatever works for you', or of imposing a

system of healing to which you are passionately dedicated. Instead, healing across cultures must start from the individual's conception of his or her world, and working through the model the clinician must strive to find mechanisms appropriate to the client's context, while keeping faith with his or her own powers of healing. Sometimes this will involve introducing new elements into the way in which individuals live their lives and understand their world. The utopian aim of the clinician working across cultures is to build healthy communities and allow them to reproduce themselves in ways that represent an adaptation to their current context. This is how 'culture' strives to survive, renewed each and every day.

## GUIDELINES FOR PROFESSIONAL PRACTICE

1. In most cultures there is a well-worn path to becoming sick. People from a different culture may not be conversant with the 'right way' to be sick. However, such a role will be facilitated by establishing good communications between patient and clinician. Clinicians should allow for more time, and perhaps more visits by the patient, before making a formal diagnosis.
2. Clinicians may well find that the practitioner placebo effect is less strong with patients from a foreign culture than with those from their own culture. Judgements about who is an effective clinician are subjective judgements (initially anyway) and usually based on faith in the clinician rather than objective data about clinical success. Clinicians should therefore be prepared for patients from a different culture to be somewhat more sceptical of their healing powers.
3. The idea of faith in clinicians and faith in treatments can be broadened further to include faith in different healers in general and faith in different types of intervention. This broader level of analysis may help clinicians appreciate how they can be liked as individuals but dismissed as therapeutic agents, or many other combinations of

reactions to them as individuals and as healers. These Faith Grids may help clinicians to think through the interactions between themselves and their patients.

4. People from different cultures will have varying expectations about the information clinicians will/should share with their patients. Benevolent diagnostic deception may seem unethical to some, while others will view the sharing of a stigmatized diagnosis as gross social irresponsibility. As clinical work is increasingly multicultural, in the sense of working with colleagues from different backgrounds, the manner in which cultural values influence clinical decision making must be considered. Likewise the patient's expectation of what will/ought to be disclosed should also be taken into account.

5. In attempting to plan for necessary treatment services, service utilization may be misleading. Some cultural groups may avoid presenting particular complaints because of the shame associated with certain problems. In such cases the role of a cultural representative may be very important in service planning.

6. Treatments are products of cultures. A particular form of psychotherapy, for instance, may strongly reflect particular cultural values. Psychotherapy may also problematize legitimate distress which arises out of the oppression of individuals of a particular culture. Therefore, sometimes, clinicians can adopt a stance to a client which makes them more a part of the problem than a part of the solution. In offering treatment, clinicians should think through what their role implies for the client's complaint.

7. Clinicians should not be hesitant about adopting approaches to treatment which emanate from another culture. However, where a power imbalance exists between cultures there is a danger of one perspective being imposed on people who have another perspective.

8. The concept of transference offers a powerful tool for understanding how the interaction between a client and clinician from different cultural backgrounds may mirror important themes concerning how these two cultures

have related to each other in the past. Clinicians, of all types, should therefore make themselves familiar with the concept of transference.

9. The 'culture-centred' approach to counselling encourages clinicians to think through abstract and hypothetical cultures, derived from the results of Hofstede's international IBM studies. This approach places culture in the foreground and risks minimizing consideration of the extent to which an individual conforms or discounts the values of his or her own culture.

10. The analysis of critical incidents may be used as an adjunct or as a more central part of a treatment intervention. The advantage of this technique is that it allows one to examine what is critical to a person and, in doing so, to derive at least some of the goals and values in their life. Such an understanding should enhance the clinician's ability to intervene in a manner that is sensitive to their client's values.

11. Intercultural therapy provides a medium for therapist and client to explore the influence of many contextual factors, including social, political, psychological, cultural, and economic factors, on the distress which may be experienced by members' of minority cultural groups. While many clinicians will feel poorly equipped to deal with such issues, an awareness that these broadly based contextual factors may contribute to mental and physical ill-health is crucial.

12. Rather than clinicians operating across cultures, it may be useful for them to consider the potential benefits of operating *through* cultures. Culture may be seen as treatment in itself. Culture can offer a system of living which marginalized groups have been displaced from, with the consequence that self-identity and self-esteem have been damaged. The benefits of 'culture as treatment' need not, however, be limited to one's own culture. Involvement with different cultures or different religious groups, which offer alternative ways of living, may also benefit some people.

# 7

# CULTURALLY SENSITIVE HEALTH SERVICES

*For practising health professionals, it is timely to take pluralism or diversity into account, to re-examine the important role culture plays in how people view and make decisions about their health. We all need periodically to re-examine our own cultural and professional biases, and to be cognisant of the current diversity in the communities we serve.*

(Mensah, 1993, p. 39)

This chapter is concerned with enhancing the cultural sensitivity of health services. It goes beyond the individuals who constitute the service to consider the systems and policies which health services must develop in order to be sensitive to the diverse needs of multicultural communities. We begin by recognizing that people's health may be served through various sectors, including the popular, folk and professional sectors. All people seeking health care bring with them their own ideas, or explanatory models, of why they are suffering. Often these models will include a pluralism of ideas which do not necessarily accord with the models of those they seek help from. The central concept of any culturally sensitive health service should be 'tolerance of pluralism'. Only through such tolerance can a health service perform its many social and therapeutic functions. We consider what barriers exist to the provision of culturally sensitive health services, and how professional training must address multicultural skills, and we then review the sort of policy initiatives which can help to create culturally sensitive health services.

## TRANSCULTURAL, CROSS-CULTURAL OR MULTICULTURAL CARE?

The way in which we care for people is influenced by the cultural and social systems in which we live. However, our modern urban communities often present a plethora of cultural and social systems. This makes the task of providing appropriate health care extremely complex and challenging. In essence, we need a way of conceptualizing what it is we want to achieve. How can the United Nations initiative of 'Health for All' actually be achieved across many different cultures? Can cultural diversity be retained while providing for equal standards of health care to be achieved? Mensah (1993) describes three perspectives on health care in the context of cultural variations.

*Transcultural* care is concerned with a comparison between cultures in terms of their caring behaviour, health and illness values, their beliefs and patterns of behaviour. The focus of this approach is on the care-giver, who has to develop expertise in understanding the groups he or she is working with in order to effectively deliver care. Thus the clinician is taught to recognize and understand the values, beliefs and practices of different cultures and in so doing is enabled to deliver care in a culturally sensitive and appropriate manner. In a sense this perspective seeks to make an anthropologist out of the clinician.

A second perspective is that of *cross-cultural* caring. The implicit assumption here is that the giver of care and the receiver of care are from different cultural backgrounds. Key issues in this approach are how well the cross-cultural bridge can be established in order to allow, for instance, a white English obstetrician to care for an Indian woman. Also of concern in this approach would be the extent to which different cultures within a community health service were utilizing the resources of the service. This has been described as 'ethnic monitoring' of health care. Related to this is the idea that cultural groups may present with different rates of particular illnesses or disorders. The cross-cultural perspective is perhaps most obviously relevant to the concerns of health service managers.

The third perspective is *multicultural* care. Multicultural care, while incorporating elements of transcultural and cross-cultural care, goes beyond these philosophies to provide both culturally appropriate and culturally sensitive care. Rather than focusing on the carer or the administration of caring services, multicultural care is concerned with the total systems of care within the community. Rather than fragmenting services, it seeks to make systems of care more effective and applicable to a broader range of people. A key element in the multicultural perspective is recognizing and addressing discrepancies between needs extant in the community and the agendas of organizations, institutions and professions which purport to serve the community. Often the conservatism and self-interest of those organizations, institutions and professions will mitigate against their recognition of the pluralism required in any health system which hopes to serve a multicultural community. It is the systemic aspect of the multicultural care philosophy which makes it particularly attractive as a model for health care.

## POPULAR, FOLK AND PROFESSIONAL SECTORS OF HEALTH CARE

Kleinman (1980) has suggested that there are three overlapping sectors of health care which constitute the health care systems of all societies. His point is that while the content of these sectors differs across cultures, their structure is the same. Essentially the health care system is structured into popular, folk and professional sectors. Each of these sectors offers a particular approach to understanding the cause of, and prescribing treatment for, illness or disorder. Each sector also defines the sufferer and the healer in its own way and has its own rules for their interaction. This model for understanding health care systems across cultures has been very influential and so we will consider each of the three sectors in turn.

## The popular sector

This is the largest sector of the health care system. However, it is important to realize that it is not formally defined as a 'sector' and does not fit into an overall planned 'health care system'. Instead, the popular sector is where everyday ideas about health and illness are discussed by 'lay', non-professional people. Healing knowledge and advice is passed on through informal discussions. This sector is where popular notions of health and illness live. It is in the popular sector that people first experience suffering. It is here that they label it and decide how to react to it. Thus family, friends, colleagues and others whom one encounters in everyday life are part of this popular sector. These people will be sources of ideas about what gives you cancer, heart disease, 'piles', 'nerves' and so on, how you know when you have them and what to do to get rid of them. The experience of suffering is often shaped through the beliefs extant in the popular sector.

As the popular sector is where suffering is first experienced, it is also this sector which usually determines whether someone seeks help from the folk or professional sectors. The popular sector is an expression of the community's beliefs about suffering and how to avoid suffering. Thus jogging, eating raw eggs, taking cold baths, wrapping up tight in the winter and not sitting in draughts are all ideas salient to health and expressed through the popular sector. It can therefore be seen that this sector has perhaps the most influential contribution to make to the prevention of suffering. The popular sector should be the vehicle for the promotion of health because it not only reflects 'popular' beliefs, but also works through community mechanisms. I have argued elsewhere (Mac-Lachlan, 1996) that health promotion, if it is to be successful, needs also to address and counteract 'anti-health promotion ideas' which are a part of the popular sector: 'There is nothing you can do to prevent AIDS', 'Enjoy life while you can' or 'AIDS is just a new word for old problems'.

The popular sector of the health care system includes: self-treatment; treatment based on the advice of family or friends, church groups, community groups, self-help groups; and seeking out other people who have experienced similar forms of suffering. Part of this sector includes the commonly accepted ways to stay healthy, and the beliefs about staying healthy will, of course, vary from culture to culture.

## Professional sector

The professional sector is composed of the organized health professions. In Europe and North America the professional health sector has become dominated by scientific medicine. The medical profession has been successful not only in terms of making other approaches to health care subservient to the medical profession ('paramedicals', 'professions allied to medicine' and so on) but also in terms of setting the health agenda. Thus 'Western' societies now tend to define, treat and evaluate suffering within a medical frame of reference. This is a substantial political 'achievement' by the medical profession when we consider the alternative models of suffering and healing available to us.

One function of professionalization is to suggest that only certain individuals should be in positions of power or have control over particular resources. This is underwritten by the assumption that only some people have the right or ability to help with certain sorts of suffering. This sense of professionalization has also been exported to less industrially developed societies. This has had some surprising and potentially challenging results for powerful professional groups in the 'West'. For instance, in Malawi, which had a 'Western'-trained medical doctor as its president for almost 30 years, there has been an attempt to develop a 'Western' system of health care. Resources have not, however, allowed for the range of professions which usually staff 'Western' hospitals.

Zomba Mental Hospital is the only major in-patient psychiatric facility in the country. Except for occasional expatriate personnel on temporary contracts, the hospital is staffed by nurses, medical assistants and medical officers. The hospital has no 'Western' qualified medical practitioners, psychiatrists, psychologists, social workers, occupational therapists or physiotherapists. In fact, only a handful of the nurses have any 'Western' training. Nonetheless, what is interesting about this situation is that, despite the lack of 'appropriate personnel' the hospital runs on a 'Western' medical model of psychiatric care; with the diagnosis, treatment (including drugs, electroconvulsive therapy and counselling), discharge and follow-up, all being undertaken under the direction of nursing staff. Such a situation would be unthinkable in most western European countries, not because nursing staff couldn't perform these same functions, but because we have been led to believe that they *shouldn't*.

The exportation and 'expertation' of the 'Western' scientific biological model, with the dominating influence of the medical profession, may have come back to haunt the 'West'. It is not just in the sphere of mental suffering that our assumptions (you might want to be seduced into calling them 'standards'!) are being challenged. School leavers with two years' subsequent specialized training are in charge of surgical operations which we may believe require 10 years of training. The point here is not to evaluate one system of health care against another (to my knowledge the effectiveness and 'value for money' of such systems has not been compared) but instead to emphasize that 'Western' health care is based on assumptions built into its system by different professional groups. There is nothing definitive or 'right' about the way they do things, rather their systems of health care, like all others, reflect the society they live in.

In 'Western' societies there are certain assumptions about who is in charge of a meeting between a health professional and a 'patient'. There are assumptions about patients 'complying' with or 'resisting' treatment and 'accepting' or 'denying' their diagnosis. It is, of course, not only patients who are victims of this system, but clinicians too. Perhaps you, like myself, have experienced a sudden loss of respect and 'magical healing power' as a result of being so 'insensitive' as to consult a book in the presence of a patient! The assumptions built into 'Western' health care systems are a direct consequence of having a professional sector based on 'expert' knowledge around the ethos of biological reductionism. Other societies have professionalized alternative approaches to healing and they too have their drawbacks. Awareness of the form and function of 'Western' health care professionalism has been the target of this section.

## Folk sector

The folk sector combines some aspects of the popular and professional sectors. It is characterized as being non-professional (in the sense of formal qualifications), non-bureaucratic (in the sense of being immediately available and not constricted by 'rules') and specialist (in the sense of folk healers having expertise in particular problems and/or treatments). The folk sector includes sacred and secular healers. While folk healers are more commonly associated with less industrialized countries, increasing internationalization has resulted in urban communities having a plethora of indigenous and foreign folk healers.

Examples of folk healers traditionally found in Europe could include, for instance, faith healers, 'mediums', gipsy fortune tellers and herbalists. It could also include a range of treatment approaches currently described as 'alternative' or 'complementary' medicine, such as homeopathy, acupuncture and hypnosis. Homeopathy, in Britain, is a particularly interesting example because, although it is seen as an 'alternative' therapy to 'modern' medicine, it was incorporated into the National Health Service, even to the extent of having specialist homeopathic hospitals. These hospitals are staffed by medically qualified practitioners who have undergone further training in homeopathy.

Increasingly, the folk sector, especially in urban areas, is incorporating healers from other traditional societies. These include 'root doctors', 'witch doctors' and a great array of spiritual healers. Folk healers from whatever culture share and articulate the social meaning of suffering as understood in their own culture. Internationalization, multiculturalism and a growing dissatisfaction with biological reductionism have combined to create an unprecedented situation. In the urban heartlands of those societies which consider themselves the most technologically and scientifically advanced in the world, we also have a wider choice of beliefs and treatments available to us than ever before. Many of these beliefs challenge the very assumptions on which technological advancement has been achieved. For instance, holism is preferred to reductionism, the involvement of family members is preferred to an 'expert' dictating the best treatment and a spiritual element to healing is sought.

## The health care matrix

Together these three sectors constitute a health care matrix which informally interlocks in some places and contradicts in others. Within each of these sectors the understanding of suffering is different and the means of removing suffering varies tremendously. Within any one society each of these sectors presents complex alternative understandings and offers a rich variety of explanatory combinations. Of course, whether the clinician is aware of them or not has no effect on their existence. As an example, I recall once treating an agoraphobic lady in Dumfries, in the borders of Scotland. In the middle of our 'session' an ambulance passed by outside with the siren wailing. The lady caught hold of the collar of her jacket and smiled apologetically while at the same time indicating that we should continue.

As we talked she kept staring out of my office window as though she was looking for something. The ambulance was long gone and the siren had faded 10 minutes ago. Finally, I asked 'Why are you holding your collar?' 'Because of the ambulance', she replied. I started to worry that I had misjudged the lady completely and responded 'Because . . . of the . . . ambulance?'. 'Oh yes, don't you know, if you see an ambulance when you're out, you must hold onto your collar until you see three dogs; otherwise it will be going to your house, the ambulance I mean.' Then she smiled warmly and said, 'Well, some people round here believe that anyway.' Ten minutes later she left the clinic still holding onto her collar and laughing a smile. Before she let go of her collar, she later told me, she saw three dogs. When she arrived home there was no ambulance there.

## EXPLANATORY MODELS

Kleinman (1980) has also addressed the issue of how people, including clinicians, explain suffering to themselves and to others. His idea is that people develop 'explanatory models' to understand their suffering. He describes this approach as 'ethnomedicine'. Essentially it is about understanding the interplay between cultural beliefs, the experience of suffering and curative methods. He argues that beliefs about illness are closely tied to beliefs about treatment. By understanding the way in which a person explains their suffering we should be able to present treatments to them more effectively. But people do not simply explain the cause of their suffering according to a model found in one of the sectors, rather each individual develops their own explanatory model for each episode of suffering, and each of these models may involve beliefs from the popular, folk and professional sectors, to a different extent. It should be emphasized that individuals' own explanatory models are not only important in the cross-cultural context, but also for understanding the illness models of people within one's own culture (Weinman *et al.*, 1996).

Clinicians also have their own explanatory models and in the professional sector these will generally relate to the substance of their professional training. However, even the explanatory models of professional clinicians will differ from one another (see Chapter 5) and some will involve aspects of popular and folk beliefs. When the clinician and the client come together, two different explanatory models are meeting. Communication involves understanding the other person's explanatory model. Sometimes the 'cognitive distance' between the models will be great and one of the parties (usually the client) will appear to modify their explanatory model and 'go along' with the understanding of the clinician.

This notion of explanatory models therefore includes the notion (albeit implicitly) that there may be some form of negotiation between the clinician and the patient. The logic for such 'negotiation' would be to come up with an explanatory model which both clinician and patient could 'work with' and which made sense to each of them. Presumably part of this idea of *making sense* is that, for instance, the cause of the problem should be related to its treatment. Thus 'cognitive distance' could be reduced by negotiation to produce a 'cognitively consistent' model.

## TOLERANCE OF PLURALISM

The ideas of popular, folk and professional systems of health care, of different explanatory models for each episode of

suffering and of a multicultural system of health care all com-
bine to present a daunting level of complexity which must
appear beyond the grasp of just about anybody! To negotiate
logically consistent explanatory models across all these levels
of complexity must surely be beyond the time, knowledge
and intellectual constraints of most of us. However, none of
this is in fact necessary if we reject the notion that *consistency*
is paramount. One problem is that in the 'Western' world
people are so convinced of the absolute necessity of being
scientific, logical and at all times consistent, that it is hard for
them to imagine how abandoning this ethos could be in any
way helpful. They are so tied to it that psychologists have
even come up with a term to describe the uncomfortable feeling which accompanies the realization of inconsistency: 'cognitive dissonance'.

Cognitive dissonance (Festinger, 1957) is experienced when
people become aware of inconsistencies in their beliefs and/
or behaviour. Since dissonance is an uncomfortable feeling, it
is argued that people (in 'Western' cultures) try to impose
consistency on their behaviours and/or beliefs in order to
create 'cognitive consonance'. This drive towards consonance
is so strong that sometimes they actually distort their beliefs
in order to make them appear to 'fit' each other. This notion of
things 'fitting' is also described by Kleinman (1980, p. 19):
'Thus, ideas about the cause of illness (as well as its pa-
thophysiology and course) are linked to ideas about practical
treatment interventions.' However, this need not be so. Ideas
about what causes an illness may be quite different from ideas
as to how to treat the same illness.

In a series of studies conducted in Malawi we have found a
lack of 'consistency' in ideas about suffering and how to alleviate it (MacLachlan & Carr, 1994a; MacLachlan, 1996a). For
instance, while people may believe in a traditional spiritual
cause for malaria, they may nonetheless prefer a modern biomedical treatment for it. We have noted this lack of consistency, or, to put it more positively, this *greater tolerance* for the

ambiguity created by acknowledging different causal models, across various illnesses in Malawi. We have also demonstrated how complex non-linear statistical regression techniques can predict apparently 'inconsistent' pluralistic beliefs about health (Carr *et al.*, 1996). If this is the case, we believe that there is a good logic behind such beliefs and that the strength of belief in any particular approach to health will be strongly influenced by the immediate context in which one is seeking help.

However, do not for a moment think that such 'inconsistency' is characteristic of only less industrialized or 'non-Western' countries. Similar 'inconsistencies' are also found in the USA, Europe and many other more industrialized regions too. In these cultures, for instance, when somebody is suffering from a virus, people often pray for them or give them a luck charm. Frequently nurses open a window in a room where someone has just died so as to 'let their soul out'. Also, people in 'Western' cultures may, for instance, take an Aspirin for a headache, but this doesn't mean that they necessarily believe that the headache was caused by a lack of Aspirin, or indeed by any other chemical deficit. On the contrary, they may ascribe its cause to overwork, guilt, heat or whatever.

The point here is not that these actions don't make any sense. They have their own therapeutic sense, but they also cross over explanatory models. Although we are often unaware of it, our ideas and behaviours regarding health are often inconsistent. This inconsistency can be viewed not as a problem but as a strength. To give it this positive connotation it may be referred to as 'cognitive tolerance'. However, it is clear that this tolerance is not restricted to any one geographical area. Its presence in the tropics is perhaps more obvious because many people living in these areas have confronted radically different systems of health care and have been able to do so without having to rubbish, or reject, all but one of them. However, this is also true elsewhere.

Bishop (1996) and colleagues working in Singapore have similarly described tolerance as an aspect of their health system. Singaporeans have access to traditional Chinese, Malay and Indian forms of healing as well as biomedical 'Western' healing. Singaporeans commonly seek help from more than one of these systems of healing at a time. Bishop (1996) has reported that, compared to North American Caucasian students, Singaporean students use a greater number of cognitive dimensions to understand disease, and synthesize 'Eastern' and 'Western' conceptions of disease to a greater extent. Jenkins *et al.* (1996) have reviewed the health-seeking behaviour of Vietnamese immigrants to the USA and concluded that although these immigrants continue to have distinctive health beliefs and practices, these aspects of their Vietnamese culture have not acted as a barrier to their seeking 'Western' health care. It would seem that they are not being 'culturally doped', or forced into one exclusive category. Instead they are being pluralistic. Nonetheless, Kleinman's assertion that beliefs about illness can influence treatment choice has also been supported by recent research (e.g. Brown & Segal, 1996). Of course, these two positions are not incompatible and once again illustrate the complex interplay between individuals, cultures and health practices.

Tolerance is a strength which clinicians also need to develop because, living in multicultural societies, we are now confronting a broader range of explanations for suffering than perhaps ever before. The recognition of different cultural explanations is also giving life to the acknowledgement of multi-sectorial explanations from within our own health care systems. Multiculturalism may have liberated us to take our own subcultural and folk perspectives on health more seriously.

The professional sector of 'Western' health care systems is hung-up on a dichotomy which other cultures do not even see as existing. 'Western' health care has extracted mind from body, even to the extent of setting up separate hospitals to deal with 'mind suffering' and 'body suffering'. Despite it being difficult to imagine one without the other, this chasm has been driven into everyday experience. This is just one example of intolerance: 'If it's not one, then it's the other, but it can't be both!' Fortunately, in many 'Western' cultures there are now growing signs of this mentality disappearing. This form of tolerance must be built on to develop a system of serving peoples' health needs which is capable of responding to their own explanatory models of suffering. This does not necessarily mean agreeing with all alternative explanations, but it does mean treating them as alternative hypotheses worthy of investigation. It also means recognizing that individuals may seek out alternative therapies because they believe that they offer something which mainstream services are lacking (Vincent & Furnham, 1996).

## FUNCTIONS OF A HEALTH CARE SYSTEM

The importance of developing tolerant health services becomes obvious when we face up to the challenge of providing health services which are culturally sensitive. A health service which reflects just one ethos of health care cannot possibly satisfy the needs of a multicultural community. Returning once again to Kleinman, we can consider five functions which a health care system should perform. First, it should be able to explain the *meaning* of suffering within the sociocultural context of the patient or client. Second, a health care system ought to create order amidst the chaos of suffering. This *ordering* may include defining which problems are most serious, which require the most urgent attention, which resources should be allocated to which problems and so on. A third function is that of *communicating*. Suffering should be classified and explained. How does the suffering relate to ideas about cause and treatment? A fourth function is to provide *healing*; that is, it should be able to alleviate suffering. Finally, the system should be capable of *managing* a range of different responses to its attempts to heal. These responses include cures, contraction of iatrogenic illnesses, worsening of the suffering people presented with and ultimately death itself.

Health care systems should also include the function of *promoting* health. Without this function we are talking about a system which cares for illness and suffering rather than one which *cares for health* (see Chapter 8). A health care system based solely on scientific and medical knowledge cannot possibly hope to perform the above functions for people who do not share this ethos. A health care system which is culturally sensitive will need to reflect different meanings, order care in different ways, comprehend different ways of communicating, provide different methods of healing, manage different responses to its attempts to heal and use different mediums to promote health.

These are indeed ambitious aims, but they are the aims of a complete system, not of every individual within the system. Appropriate management of the system can provide the tolerance and plurality discussed above. Before describing some of the organizational features of a culturally sensitive health care system, I would like to focus on some of the misconceptions which can discourage individuals from embracing such an approach.

## BARRIERS TO MULTICULTURAL HEALTH CARE

As health service providers have become more aware of the demands of multicultural communities an array of exciting initiatives have been launched to met such demands. However, a number of lores (as in folklore), or myths, have also characterized some of the thinking on developing multicultural community health services. In this section we consider some of these barriers, the rationales behind them, and how they might be overcome. Some of this discussion is based on Masi's (1993) excellent paper on 'Multicultural health'.

## 'Positive discrimination is necessary'

It is now common to see advertisements for health or welfare positions which specify preference for applicants from a particular cultural minority. This is called 'positive discrimination', where there is an attempt to encourage applicants of a certain cultural background. There may be several reasons for this. Often cultural minorities are under-represented, and so in order to provide health and welfare services more commensurate with the community they seek to serve, people from such minority cultures are targeted in advertising campaigns. However, unless those responsible for selection are seeking specified ratios of, for instance, white Germans, Turks, Arabs, Chinese, simply increasing the number of non-white-Germans may result in an equally unrepresentative service. This sort of positive discrimination has led to the now common quip that 'If you're white, male, middle aged and middle class, then you're soon going to be unemployable!' Of course this is an exaggeration based on a reduction in the employment privileges previously enjoyed by this section of 'Western' society. No doubt it also reflects some fear of, and resistance to, changing the privileged position of a powerful cultural group.

Many would argue that positive discrimination should take place at the level of opportunity rather than the level of selection. Thus different cultural groups should be given equal access to resources, including education. Members of the minority groups would then work their way through the system on the basis of merit rather than cultural preference. The drawback with this notion is that minority cultures, for instance newly arrived immigrants, may not be able (because of language, economic or social reasons) to take advantage of available resources to the same extent that indigenous people can. The other drawback is that a 'work your way through the system approach' will necessarily have a time-lag built into it before it bears fruit. Nonetheless, it may be that for workers from minority cultures to be accepted as equals among their co-workers they need to be seen as having equal merit.

Positive discrimination is not necessarily beneficial, in the long run, either to the individual selected or to the minority cultural group being served.

## 'Like should treat like'

Related to the idea of positive discrimination is the idea that clinicians ought to be of the same cultural background as the people they are helping. Again there is a good rationale to this. It is argued that only a clinician of the same cultural heritage as the client can be sensitive to and understand the full cultural context of the client's suffering. However, several objections to this can be raised. First, simply because two people are from the same culture does not mean that they are able to understand each other's social context. They may be from different subcultures. Thus a French medical doctor from a well-off family who was educated at exclusive private schools, as well as university, may be no better able to empathize with the despair of a single parent housewife from a 'rough' Paris housing estate, than might an Indian doctor from a poor area of Bombay.

A second objection to the 'like should treat like' philosophy is that it fails to take account of the complexities of the therapeutic relationship. The key element in the selection of an appropriate clinician should be their ability to work effectively as a clinician. While this ability can surely be tempered by the context in which one works, it should not be overshadowed by it. Sometimes a clinician's interest in people from a different culture will provide the motivation to perform very well. The 'like should treat like' philosophy thus has some points in its favour and some points against it.

## 'All or Nothing'

This attitude implies that if we cannot tailor health care to the idiosyncratic needs of each culture represented in a community then we should not tailor it to anyone. Certainly no individual practitioner can hope to understand how, perhaps, 20 different cultures relate to health and welfare, but it is not necessary that he or she should, if we can utilize the multicultural approach described above. This is concerned with developing *systems* of health care to accommodate the diversity of cultures which are the reality of many modern urban communities. It does not require each practitioner to be acquainted equally well with each culture; instead it requires a health system to have the capacity to deal equally well with the health and welfare problems which can be presented by members of different cultures within the community.

The approach I have advocated confers the potential for understanding how different cultures see health. It does this by focusing on the process of gaining information rather than on the content of the information (see Chapter 2). To provide lots of 'facts' on Chinese ideas about health is simply to encourage fruitless stereotyping about what an ill Chinese person 'should' think is wrong with him. The essence of cultural sensitivity in the clinic is to learn about culture as it impacts on the person who needs one's help. This perspective always reminds us of the enormous variation between individuals of the same culture.

## ' "Culture" can be used to justify anything.'

This barrier relates to an excessive degree of 'cultural relativism'. Cultural relativism is the doctrine that everything is relative and that if you truly understand a culture then you will also appreciate the function of behaviours which might otherwise appear cruel, discriminatory or offensive. It is then extrapolated from this that one should not criticize the behaviour of people from another culture. Consequently, people can use their culture to justify whatever they like: 'You don't understand my culture . . . and you shouldn't criticize what you don't understand . . . just because its different from your culture. . . .'

Such an extreme position need not be accepted. Presumably all cultures have some bad things about them, as well as some good things. For instance, it could be argued that it is part of the Irish 'culture' that Protestants and Catholics should dislike each other. Few would see this as a good characteristic and few, I believe, would object to finding ways to alleviate such sectarian tensions. If this was successfully done then indeed one could argue that the Irish culture had been changed, or interfered with. Clearly the same argument can be used with other cultures. The laws of a society will also determine what is acceptable and what is unacceptable. Occasionally these laws may take into account cultural differences (for instance, in Britain Sikh motorcyclists need not wear a helmet over their turbans) but in general they demand similar behaviour from across cultural groups. Thus the law can always be used as a recourse.

Recall the case study of 'cultural asylum' concerning the culturally sanctioned initiation ceremony which Yoruba girls experience. Rightly or wrongly, the laws of one society were used to prevent the customs of another society being practised. The cultural relativism argument fails to recognize that cultures are dynamic, ever-changing, social systems. They are not historical artefacts to be preserved at all costs. For a culture to 'survive' it must adapt to its contemporary environment.

## 'Cultural sensitivity: either you have it or you don't.'

It is often thought that cultural sensitivity is a matter of personality type or communication ability. While some people are certainly more empathic and have better communication skills than others, cultural sensitivity is an ability which can be developed through training. Many large multinational companies now require their top executives to undergo cultural sensitivity training before letting them loose on clients in foreign countries. This requirement is not simply a philosophical commitment to a multicultural ethos, rather it is in recognition that people can be taught to interact more effectively with people from cultures different to their own. The same is certainly true with health professionals. This is especially so when we consider how culture can influence the cause, experience, expression and treatment of suffering.

## Summary

These, then, are just some of the objections which are sometimes raised to the provision of multicultural health services. It is important to appreciate how they are weak objections. Health care professionals *can* be made more culturally aware, and can develop skills which will increase their effectiveness as clinicians. In the next section we consider some of the ways in which this can be achieved.

# PROFESSIONAL TRAINING

Unfortunately many health professions continue to give scant attention to cultural sensitivity in their training requirements. Cultural sensitivity is perhaps seen as the 'software' of clinical skills rather than its 'hardware', which is perhaps thought of as being the factual knowledge and concrete skills generally assessed in professional examinations. However, the importance of cultural awareness extends beyond interpersonal and communication skills into the core of clinical practice. First of all let us consider how to conceptualize cultural sensitivity in clinical practice.

## Conceptual awareness

Rogler and colleagues (1987) have described a pyramidal framework for conceptualizing clinical innovations in providing culturally sensitive mental health services. Their framework need not be restricted to mental health and can be applied to all health services. At the bottom of their framework is **increasing the accessibility of treatment** to cultural minorities. In practice this may mean reducing the gap between professional and subcultural perceptions of health problems and needs. It is also likely to involve the modification of referral procedures. For instance, consultation with and/or inclusion of traditional cultural healers may help in this. It may also involve confronting linguistic barriers (see below).

The next level up the pyramid is the **selection of treatments to fit particular cultures**. In terms of modality of treatment this may, for instance, mean that physicians will work with families rather than with individuals. For psychotherapists it could mean giving more emphasis to interpreting dreams than they would usually do. For psychiatrists it may mean appreciating that not all cultural groups respond to drugs in the same way (Casimir & Morrison, 1993). In addition, it has been reported that the propensity to take home-made remedies in preference to prescribed medication is influenced by culture, poverty status, education, the severity of the problem, as well as the perceived costs and benefits of home-made remedies (Brown & Segal, 1996). Within any one particular cultural group the selection of treatments may also involve distinguishing between those who are acculturated (or pluralistic) to the extent of being able to accept conventional treatments and those who wish treatments that are traditional in their culture of origin.

At the top of the pyramid is **modification of treatments to fit particular cultures**. In essence, this is an extension of modifying treatments to fit the individual. It assumes that some treatment modalities may be more effective in some cultures than in others. As opposed to selecting the most appropriate treatment, this approach calls for the development of new treatments. It is clearly the highest level of delivering culturally sensitive health services and deserves the considerable research interest which it is now attracting. Appreciating this sort of 'compartmentalization' is an important aspect of professional training (Ho, 1985).

## Mechanisms for encouraging cultural sensitivity in training

Casimir and Morrison (1993) have suggested various mechanisms for ensuring that cultural sensitivity is given a high profile in professional training. Unfortunately, I believe that many of these would be difficult to manage and/or very unpopular with staff. One notion is to offer salary differentials for staff who are 'culturally competent'. Such competence would be treated like a specialization within the profession's domain. This would require making culture competence teachable and measurable so that it could constitute an aspect of certification or performance appraisal.

Another idea has been the use of paid 'minority mentors' who teach and supervise clinicians who are working with minority groups as part of their training. Related to this is the idea of pairing off clinicians with 'traditional' healers from the client's cultural group to work as co-therapists. Traditional co-therapists will have a knowledge of culture-specific syndromes and treatments from which the 'contemporary' clinician may gain.

While each of the above methods of transferring skills of cultural competence may be of some benefit, modifying the usual approach to professional training may also be important. The training programmes of most health professions do not acknowledge that health beliefs and practices do vary across cultural groups. Instead, professional training seeks to achieve competence in universal principles. An emphasis on understanding the influence of socioeconomic status, gender and culture would better prepare clinicians to be sensitive to the needs of minority groups.

## Defining culturally competent training

Bernal and Castro (1994) recently reviewed the extent to which clinical psychology training programmes in the United States prepared trainees for clinical practice and research with minority cultural groups. They compared the results of their survey with those of a previous survey, also carried out by Bernal 10 years earlier. They reported a number of positive developments: the number of programmes offering modules on minority cultures had increased; the use of resource people from minority cultural groups (e.g. health professionals, community workers, lay people) had increased; the use of community mental health agencies serving minority cultural populations, as training placements, had also increased. However, in contrast to this: 39 per cent of clinical training programmes still had no minority-related courses; 40 per cent of programmes did not use off-campus clinical settings serving minority cultural groups; and one-third of programmes had no faculty (staff) member from a cultural minority. Bernal and Castro therefore concluded that the results revealed a 'mixed picture of progress'.

Bernal and Castro suggest that courses which train for 'cultural proficiency' are proactive and may be characterized as:

(a) having a high regard and respect for cultures;
(b) including a knowledge base which exposes all students (i.e. not optional modules) to a standard cultural content that relates directly to basic clinical competencies (e.g. assessment) and provides opportunity for in-depth understanding of specific health issues relating to minorities through speciality courses;
(c) continuing efforts to add to the knowledge base of culturally competent practice through the development and evaluation of new therapeutic and prevention approaches *based on culture*;
(d) planning and coordinating links between didactic course work and practical field experiences;

(e) paying careful attention to the dynamics of group dif-
    ferences in the training setting and in research and prac-
    tice; and

(f) providing for a continuous infusion of cultural knowl-
    edge and resources through regular evaluation of the
    training curriculum.

While these criteria for culturally competent training programmes have been developed with reference to clinical psychology doctorates, they are broad enough to be applicable to
most health professional training programmes. The extent to
which such initiatives are proposed, encouraged and taken up
often depends on the context in which health services are
provided. Health care policy and administration can therefore
be very influential through creating a receptive environment.

## HEALTH CARE POLICY AND ADMINISTRATION

When providing guidelines for the clinician it is important to
remember the systems and contexts within which individual
clinicians work. Community health care can be made
culturally sensitive by incorporating certain ideas into the
overall policies of community services. We end this chapter
by considering some policy guidelines which can drive
culturally sensitive community health services. In doing so
we draw on the policy document of Ontario Province, in Canada, which has well-developed guidelines in this regard.

## Who is in the community?

This issue relates mainly to the demographic 'shape' of the
community and would include information on age, sex, education, socioeconomic status in addition to the cultural mix
within the community. The history of immigration into the
community is also an important consideration as cultural
groups which have recently immigrated may have different

health needs from those groups who are longer established. In addition to this, some cultural groups will present with health requirements quite different from either the local population or other immigrants. An example of this would be sickle-cell anaemia being much more common in West Africans than in other cultural groups. Thus demographic profiles must reflect cultural variations if they are to be of any use in planning a service to meet the needs of the community.

## What is on paper?

The power of the written word is often overlooked by clinicians focused on action at the 'coal face' of health service delivery. Yet a commitment in writing, in the dullest looking policy statement, can be an essential pivot for action. It is increasingly common these days for organizations within the health sector to issue 'mission statements'. These are essentially statements concerning what the service is trying to achieve and how it is trying to do it: for example, 'We are committed to delivering quality health services to the population of . . . by focusing on the needs of individuals and families.' The mission statement is very important because the organization is often run to achieve the aims described in it. Such statements should therefore make reference to cultural issues.

Whether through the mission statement or other strategy documents, certain principles should be documented. First and foremost there should be a recognition of responsibility to provide health services which are equally accessible to all members of the community, including (explicitly) minority culture groups. Having equal accessibility is, however, not enough. All members of the community could have equal (and plentiful) 'access' to services for the elderly on the one hand and equal (and no) access to services catering for people with sickle-cell anaemia on the other. Thus health services must also be equitable in terms of providing equally for the health needs of each cultural group.

## What are the mechanisms for empowerment?

Cultural groups within a community can be empowered by having their views fairly represented and by allowing for their participation in decision-making processes. This means having people from minority groups as members of the committees and boards which govern health provision and draw up health strategy. Sometimes, where a board is elected, minority groups will be under-represented (almost by definition). In this case, having 'advisers' to the board can ensure that minority groups are still consulted as part of the decision-making process. Seeking feedback and surveying customer satisfaction are other ways of accessing minority opinion and this should be done on a continuous basis.

## What operational contingencies are there?

Communication is one of the most obvious difficulties which a clinician faces in trying to understand the suffering of someone from a different culture. Empathy and accuracy are essential to the therapeutic encounter. While having someone translate between the clinician and the client is never an ideal solution, it is often the only realistic way to communicate where neither speaks the other's language well. Policy statements should specify the languages for which translation will be provided. In addition to this, policy statements should also specify how health services will be sensitive to different cultural norms and values. This must include religious and dietary considerations.

## Is cultural sensitivity reflected in personnel policies and practices?

We have already discussed the importance of cultural minorities being recruited into community health services. Ideally the staff of community health services will be representative of the cultural mix within their community. However, the reality is that this ideal may be some way off for many communities, especially those with recently arrived immigrants. Furthermore, just because a community health service has a staff profile which reflects the cultural groups within its catchment area, this does not imply that the service is in any way culture sensitive. The management of personnel may still reflect biases in practices such as performance appraisal and selection for promotion.

Regarding the provision of health services to the community, each clinician, ancillary worker and manager should be required to undergo training in cultural awareness and sensitivity. Being a member of a minority group in no way exempts one from cultural insensitivity! Staff development courses should avoid the 'making *us* more sensitive to *their* needs' ethos and incorporate instead an approach which 'makes everybody more sensitive to the needs of different sectors of the community'. This latter ethos fits well with awareness of the needs of other minority groups such as people with physical handicaps, blind people, those suffering with schizophrenia or alcoholism—all of whom also have special needs requiring the sensitive provision of services.

## How is cultural sensitivity evaluated?

There are many ways in which the cultural sensitivity of health services could be evaluated. One approach would be to establish whether the health needs of different cultural groups were being served to an equivalent extent. Evaluation will always be a delicate issue and even though the focus may be on evaluating a service, individual clinicians will inevitably feel that they are themselves being assessed. However, while evaluation must address the extent to which an organization is meeting its operational and strategic objects, it must also have a 'bottom up' component. That is, the grass roots concerns of the people being served should also influence the sort of evaluation undertaken.

Customer 'satisfaction' surveys may be one way of evaluating the cultural sensitivity of health services. Other forms of assessment and feedback might include special advisory committees, soliciting comments from community organizations which represent minority cultural groups, or seeking advice from 'cultural healers' concerning the extent to which they believe the needs of their own culture are being met. It should always be remembered that often minority groups coming to 'Western' countries experience their 'new' health service to be 'more advanced' than the one they left behind. They may therefore feel that criticism would be either inappropriate or poorly received. In this sense getting accurate feedback from cultural minorities may be especially difficult. In this circumstance a strong argument can be made for the use of personal interviews (preferably by people from the same culture) as opposed to questionnaire assessment. A skilled interviewer will be better able to give the client 'permission' to be frank about how well his or her health needs are being met.

## SUMMARY

The multicultural care philosophy of providing flexible systems of care which may be applied across different cultures has certain advantages over the transcultural and cross-cultural approaches. A multicultural framework within the professional sector may also be more able to accommodate contributions from the popular and folk sectors towards providing comprehensive health care. It is always important to remember that people have different explanatory models of suffering, not just across different health sectors but also within each health sector. One of the central features of culturally sensitive health services must therefore be tolerance of pluralism. If a health care system is to perform its many social functions then that system must allow for different interpretations of health, illness and suffering. The complexity of the challenge of providing culturally sensitive systems of health care has led to some erroneous assumptions which have acted as barriers to their development. A still significant problem, however, is the low priority given to cultural issues in the training programmes of many health professions. There is much that can be done to promote cultural sensitivity at the level of policy and administration. Rather than addressing cultural issues in isolation they should be seen as part of a broader drive towards serving the needs of minority groups within the community.

## GUIDELINES FOR PROFESSIONAL PRACTICE

1. Clinicians should adopt a multicultural perspective in their work. This perspective goes beyond the comparison of different cultures, or communication in the clinician–client relationship, to consider the total system of care within a community. It can be especially important for community clinicians to understand where they 'fit in' to the overall system of providing for a multicultural service.
2. Professionally qualified clinicians are but one part of the health care which is available to people. The popular and folk sectors also have an important influence on health behaviour. Clinicians should try to establish the extent to which individuals draw from these different sectors in deciding on their health-related behaviour. Even clinicians working in a monocultural context will encounter influential beliefs, emanating from the popular and folk sectors, which may be significantly different to their own professional beliefs.
3. One of the predominant characteristics of 'Western' health care is that it has become heavily professionalized. This makes health care professionals suspicious and dismissive of people who have not been 'legitimized' by similar training. Consequently, traditional cultural healers may not be taken seriously simply because they do not conform to our cultural expectations of (usually) academic achievement. Indigenous healers may be dismissed in the same fashion.
4. While is seems reasonable to believe that beliefs about the cause of a problem and beliefs about the solution to a problem should be on the same explanatory dimensions, this

may not be the case. One of the keystones of a multicultural approach to health is for clinicians to show tolerance of pluralism. A good deal of research now supports the contention that many lay people are able to tolerate more than one explanation for a disease or disorder. This is likely to be especially so in multicultural communities which present a diversity of explanations for certain problems. The clinician who precludes all explanatory models except his or her own, is likely to be seen as narrow minded, defensive and conceited.

5. Health care systems can be understood as fulfilling a number of different functions, such as explaining the meaning of suffering, being a medium of communication about suffering and providing healing. Individual clinicians or groups working together might benefit by assessing how well they provide for each of the functions outlined in this chapter, especially within a multicultural context.

6. A number of barriers to multicultural health care exist which can be characterized as myths. These include the belief that positive discrimination is necessary, that like should treat like, that 'culture' can be used to justify anything, and so on. Clinicians should examine some of the assumptions, or folklore, which may have built up through their own experience of working in a multicultural environment. They should ask 'What is the evidence for this assumption?'

7. Those who train health professionals have much work to do. Training should include not only conceptual awareness of multicultural issues, but also mechanisms for enhancing cultural competence and exposure to clinical problems occurring in cultural contexts different to that of the trainee. Training courses can uniquely legitimize multiculturalism by requiring this perspective through examinations and practical placements.

8. Health care policy makers and administrators also have a crucial contribution to enhancing truly multicultural health care. For they are the people who set the context through which front-line clinicians operate. Appropriate policies and structures can do much to facilitate multiculturalism.

# 8

# PROMOTING HEALTH ACROSS CULTURES

In this chapter we consider the concepts of health promotion, risk reduction, and the prevention of disease and disorder from a cultural perspective. In the more industrialized countries, the public health has been improving throughout the last century and much of this improvement can be attributed to improved living conditions rather than to biomedical innovations. However, access to good public health services is not equal and minority cultural groups, who often occupy the lower socio-economic strata, have less exposure to, and therefore opportunity to benefit from, health-promoting initiatives. Here we will pay particular attention to recent recommendations for preventing mental disorders which incorporate the idea of 'cultural competence'. To give a more concrete example we return to the problem of depression, critically examining efforts to prevent depression and promote mental health across cultural minorities. We also examine the possibility that different cultures encourage different cognitions about the self and that some cultures can predispose its members to certain disorders, such as depression. This raises the possibility that culture can be a risk factor in itself. Subcultures may also constitute risk factors and to illustrate this we consider how disordered communities are being created by rural depopulation and international legislation. We conclude that health promotion may not be something which can be accommodated within existing social systems, but that, in some cases, it may only work through changing social systems.

# THE HEALTH PROMOTION MOVEMENT

Over the last century the leading causes of death in the more industrialized countries have changed dramatically. While in the 1900s pneumonia/influenza, tuberculosis and diarrhoea were the most common causes of death, cancers and diseases of the heart and cardiovascular system are now the most common causes of death. This decrease in infectious diseases as causes of death has gone hand in hand with a lengthening in average life expectancy from 40–50 years in 1900 to over 70 years by the late 1980s. For a species which has been evolving for thousands of years, this flight into longevity is outstandingly dramatic and a testimony to the benevolent potential of modern life. However, what has brought about this dramatic change?

The rate of innovation in biomedical technology has similarly increased exponentially over the past 100 years. From Alexander Fleming's accidental discovery of penicillin in 1929 we are now, on a daily basis, striding through the genetic landscape of humanity with the remarkable Human Genome Project which aims to give us a complete 'map' of the genetic make-up of *Homo sapiens*. That which was once sacred is now science. CAT (Computerized Axial Tomography), MRI (Magnetic Resonance Imaging) and PET (Positron Emission Tomography) are modern imaging devices which allow us to look inside the human brain as it works away. Souls and minds have been subverted by high-tech Peeping Toms. 'Keyhole surgery' describes a degree of surgical precision undreamt of by nineteenth-century surgeons whose trade was so base and butcher-like that they were not even dignified by the title 'doctor'. Today surgeons can 'cut' into internal organs without the need of a knife and without the blemish of a scar. We are indeed fortunate to live in such an age, where possibly our greatest challenge is to keep up with, and keep financing, the unsatiable fast forwarding of biotechnology.

It is therefore perhaps only 'common sense' to make a link between the remarkable increase in life expectancy on the one hand and the remarkable increase in biotechnological sophistication on the other. What is surprising is that such a link is by no means clear. Figure 8.1 shows how the rate of death across a range of infectious diseases fell between 1900 and 1973 in the USA. It also indicates the point at which biotechnology presented an effective means of combating each disease. This illustrates that the decline in death rate cannot fully be accounted for by biotechnological innovations. If this is so, then what can account for this improvement in health? While there is some debate about the relative contribution of different factors, improved living conditions, reduced malnutrition, improved sanitation of food and water and better systems of sewage disposal can probably take much of the credit for longer life. These factors, while not necessarily inconsistent with biotechnological innovation, are primarily concerned with the prevention of disease rather than with the high-tech treatment of disease.

This public health approach to disease emphasizes the importance of preventing the conditions which cause disease. This notion of prevention is not, however, restricted to large-scale public health interventions such as improving sewage management or water supply. Psychological factors in the form of individual's health-related behaviours can have an equally dramatic effect on mortality. What about your own mortality? How many of the following health-related practices do you engage in?

1. Sleeping seven to eight hours daily.
2. Eating breakfast almost every day.
3. Never or rarely eating between meals.
4. Currently being at or near prescribed height-adjusted weight.
5. Never smoking cigarettes.
6. Moderate or no use of alcohol.
7. Regular physical activity.

Before reading any further make sure you have a realistic idea of the number of these you can truly lay claim to. In 1965

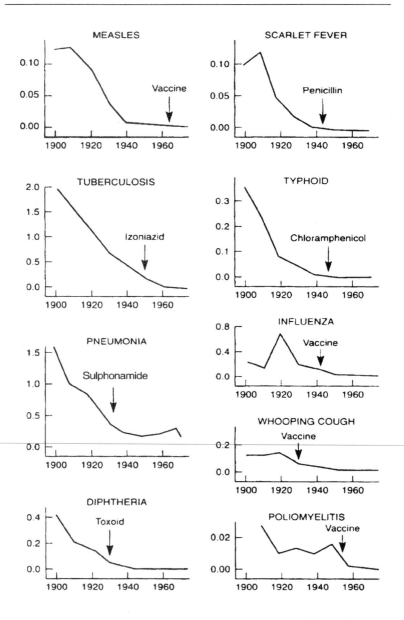

**Figure 8.1:** Standard death rate (per 100 population) for nine common infectious diseases in relation to specific medical measures in the USA (1900–1973) (reproduced from McKinlay and McKinlay, 1981, with permission)

Belloc and Breslow (1972) asked the same question of almost 7,000 people who formed a representative sample of Alamede County in California. At the time of the survey, those in better health claimed to be engaging in more of the above health practices. However, the most interesting results came from their follow-up studies. Figure 8.2 shows the proportion of this sample surviving 5½ years later as a function of the number of health behaviours reported in the original survey, their age and sex. Once again, the effects are clear and dramatic. Those people who reported engaging in a greater number of the seven health-related practices had a greater probability of being alive 5½ years later. For men this effect was particularly strong in the 55–75 age range. The positive relationship between these rather innocuous, easily executed, health behaviours and subsequent mortality also held up in a subsequent 9½ years follow-up study (see Breslow & Enstrom, 1980). How many of these seven health practices did you endorse? Your future is in your present.

While biotechnological innovation can greatly enhance our capacity for treating life-threatening conditions, improvements in public health provision and the performance of simple health-related behaviours can also play a dramatic role in lengthening life. These preventive factors should contribute not only to the quantity of life but also to the quality of life. Preventive interventions are often directed at the context of people's lives, at the circumstances they live in and at the way in which they behave. Once again, it is cultures and communities which are the vehicles for the social context through which people live. Different contexts present different threats to health and welfare, but they will also present different opportunities for intervention and different barriers to interventions. Thus effective preventive interventions in one context should not be assumed to be transferable across cultures, whether these cultures are in different parts of the world or different parts of the same city. The complexity of preventive intervention across cultures has recently been recognized in the field of mental health, to which we now turn.

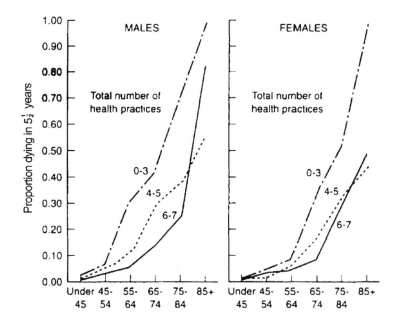

**Figure 8.2:** Age-specific mortality rates by number of health practices and gender (reproduced from Matarazzo, 1984, with permission)

## PREVENTING MENTAL DISORDERS

At the request of the United States Congress, the Institute of Medicine produced a multidisciplinary report on *Reducing Risks for Mental Disorders* (Mrazek & Haggerty, 1994). This is an important document because it claims to speak authoritatively on the development of preventive interventions for mental disorders. One of the issues (briefly) dealt with in the report is how practitioners need to develop 'a set of skills and a perspective that have become commonly known as cultural competence' (p. 391).

*Cultural sensitivity* and *cultural competence* are conceptualized as existing along a continuum. Cultural sensitivity is about being aware of relevant issues. It therefore concerns an intellectual assimilation of relevant information. Cultural sensitivity is seen as necessary, but not sufficient, for cultural competence. At the other end of the continuum, cultural competence requires personal experience of working with different cultures in order to be able to achieve a practical and appropriate match between intervention strategies and the cultural context of the intervention. Here the benchmark is not an intellectual fit but a pragmatic collaboration, wherein the targets of the intervention will feel some ownership over the strategies employed and some real benefits from their participation.

## Criteria for the prevention of mental disorders

The multidisciplinary 'Committee on the Prevention of Mental Disorders' which produced this report highlighted 10 points relating to the prevention of mental disorders where particular attention should be given to cultural competence. I will now give a brief interpretation of these points, several of which overlap and run into each other and are, at times, ambiguous.

### Forging relationships between researchers and community

There is a real danger that much of the drive for preventing mental disorders will come from distant government ministries or academic institutions, rather than from the communities which will be the sites for intervention programmes. Such a 'Top-Down' approach must be avoided at all costs. Communities must be allowed to define their own needs, their own targets and their own outcome measures. As such, health services will have to link into the appropriate extant networks of authority and communication in a given culture. Collaboration will have to be actual and active rather than a passive aspiration. For the health practitioner this may mean accepting a sharing of power, authority and knowledge with appropriate community members. Thus the content and process of intervention are likely to be the product of a negotiation process between the beliefs and aspirations of the community and those of the health practitioner(s).

### Identifying risks, mechanisms, triggers and processes

Different cultural groups are likely to differ in what constitutes the risks, mechanisms, triggers and processes for mental disorder. Thus in different cultures different causes may result in the same disorder or the same cause may result in different disorders. For instance, among the Hopi (Indians of North America) there is an increased risk of suicide among the children of parents who enter into traditionally disapproved marriages (for example, between tribes). The children are stigmatized by the labelling of their parents as deviant, and therefore encounter a series of accompanying social stressors. The same may be true of other cultural groups where colour, sect or religion presents a social barrier, the transgression of which may have harmful effects on the children of such marriages. The point here is that the specific social norms and lores of different cultures can be expected to impact through unique risks, mechanisms, triggers and processes on the health and welfare of its members.

### Employing relevant theoretical frameworks

A relevant theoretical framework for a particular community will be one which the members of that community employ in their daily living. The way in which health and welfare are understood does not only vary across cultures but also within cultures. Health practitioners may, for instance, be absolutely convinced by the theory that malaria is transmitted by the biting of mosquitoes, while those who are frequently bitten can easily dismiss it. Their own theory may be built on the immediacy of their own experience: 'Why, when we are bitten ten times a day, should one mosquito bite, one day, cause such a dramatic reaction?' 'And even if a mosquito is some-how involved in the process, then why must it be such an arbitrary event, a biological game of Russian roulette, without any social meaning or significance?' 'Why rush out and buy mosquito nets when mosquitoes are only one vector at the disposal of malevolent spirits?' 'Why not instead go to the source of the problem and appease the spirits?' Part of the challenge for the health practitioner is to employ a theoretical framework which makes enough sense to those they are try-ing to assist—*sense* being related to understanding a culture's way of existing in the world – while at the same time being able to deliver actionable ideas for practical interventions which will produce beneficial results.

### Preparing the content, format and delivery of preventive interventions

In the light of what has been stated through the three pre-vious points, it follows that there is a need to ensure that the way in which preventive interventions are undertaken em-brace rather than alienate cultural vehicles of communication. There needs to be a constant process of checking and recheck-ing the appropriateness of content, format and delivery of interventions. One practical way in which this can be done is to pay close attention to the lessons to be learnt from pilot work and pretesting.

### Adopting appropriate narrative structures and discourse

Who is willing to discuss what, with whom, and in what way? There are as many answers to this as there are customs of communication. Barriers to communication within a culture can include age, gender and status. For instance, issues about AIDS may be more openly discussed in single-sex groups than in mixed-sex groups. Particular metaphors may be used by some subcultures but be quite meaningless to others: 'My plates of meat are aching', 'I am feeling low', 'I'm so tired I could fall asleep on a clothesline'! The essential point here is that across cultures not only do the rules of engagement differ, but the way in which you engage another person also differs.

### Tapping critical decision-making processes

The way in which decisions are made varies across cultures. In some cases one person decides, in others a council of elders may decide, while in some cultures the whole community or even the whole nation may be involved in the decision-making process. Some cultures invest authority in child rearing to mothers, others to fathers, others to maternal uncles and so on. There is no one way of doing anything! Interventions which do not take these variations into account are unlikely to meet with success.

### Determining points of intervention leverage

The decision-making processes within any culture will influence where those points of intervention are which can have greatest influence. Often the greatest leverage will be through recognized leaders; however, this need not exclude other conduits of change, as described in the next section.

### Recognizing social networks and natural helpers

Within a cultural community there are also other types of authority and influence working through a variety of formal and informal social networks. Thus there may be several important points of leverage and conduits through which to address interventions. Ignoring an influential group or an influential individual down the 'intervention line,' and in doing so undermining that person's position, may be costly. Many cultures socially sanction certain types of people to do certain types of job. In Ireland, a well-off middle-class family may advertise for an au pair girl to help out with the house work, and to look after the children, in exchange for 'bed and board' and an opportunity to learn English. However, to advertise for an au pair boy, is definitely not the done thing! In Ireland foreign girls, but not foreign boys, are socially sanctioned for this task. It is important to recognize and empower the community's inherent social networks and 'natural helpers' in any intervention roles.

### Seeking fidelity of implementation

This reads a bit like a 'jargon statement'. It refers to the desire which researchers have for real-world interventions to 'keep faith' with the models they are predicated upon. In reality, applying interventions across different cultures will require a degree of flexibility and adaptation of the methods used. The researcher's concern is that these modifications do not change the underlying basic nature of the intervention variables. The practitioner's concern may be focused more on whether 'it' works, rather than specifying exactly what the 'it' is. However, the researcher only values a positive outcome if he or she can attribute it to specific intervention variables. Without knowing what aspects of an intervention package have been responsible for a positive outcome, it is impossible to predict the success of a similar intervention in another context, or even in the same context, but at another time.

### Replicating interventions across diverse and changing populations

While seeking fidelity of implementation is about being true to a model of intervention, the present point emphasizes the practical difficulties, not only in standardization, but in matching the style of intervention across such a broad range of knowledge, skills, language, linguistic ability, etc., that exists in many modern multicultural urban centres. For instance, it is estimated that the dozen or more distinct Asian-American groups—including Japanese, Chinese, Koreans, Vietnamese and Cambodians—speak more than 75 different languages. Furthermore, depending on the particular group and how long they have been resident in North America, between one-quarter and three-quarters do not speak English 'very well'. Such practical communication problems are certainly a challenge to those implementing intervention programmes.

### Summary

The above points are therefore a sort of 'top 10' listing of salient issues in the process of prevention across cultures. Table 8.1 describes a series of risk factors for the development of psychological disorders. In previous chapters we have already noted that many of these risk factors may be particularly pertinent to minority cultural groups who are often marginalized socially, economically and politically. To think through how these factors apply to a particular disorder, and bearing in mind what has previously been said about depression, let us consider which risk factors are hypothesized to predispose to depression.

## Risk factors for depression

The Committee on the Prevention of Mental Disorders' review of the literature suggests the following five risk factors for the development of depression:

1. *Having a parent or other close biological relative with a mood disorder.* It is suggested that the risk of developing depression becomes greater the larger is the proportion of genes shared with a 'mood-disordered individual'. Thus if your mother suffered with depression you would be more likely to develop depression yourself than if your uncle was the closest relation to you who had suffered with depression. It is argued that the strength of hereditary influence diminishes with less severe (subclinical) mood problems and that, even for the more severe disorders, the mechanisms of genetic transmission remain unclear.
2. *Having a severe stressor.* Examples of such stressors include a loss, divorce, marital separation, unemployment, job

**Table 8.1:** Some generic risk factors for the development of psychological disorder

| *Family circumstances* | *Ecological context* |
|---|---|
| Low social class | Neighbourhood disorganization |
| Family conflict | Racial injustment |
| Mental illness in the family | Unemployment |
| Large family size | Extreme poverty |
| Poor bonding to parents | |
| Family disorganization | *Constitutional handicaps* |
| Communication deviance | Perinatal complications |
| | Sensory disabilities |
| *Emotional difficulties* | Organic handicaps |
| Child abuse | Neurochemical imbalance |
| Apathy or emotional blunting | |
| Emotional immaturity | *Interpersonal problems* |
| Stressful life events | Peer rejection |
| Low self-esteem | Alienation and isolation |
| Emotional dyscontrol | |
| | *Skill development delays* |
| *School problems* | Subnormal intelligence |
| Academic failure | Social incompetence |
| Scholastic demoralization | Attentional deficits |
| | Reading disabilities |
| | Poor word skills and habits |

Reproduced from Coie *et al.* (1993). Copyright © 1993 by the American Psychological Association. Reprinted with permission.

dissatisfaction, a chronic physical disorder, a traumatic experience or a learning disorder. Such stressors, especially when cumulating over time, are associated with an increased risk for a range of mental disorders including depression.

3. *Having low self-esteem, a sense of low self-efficacy, and a sense of helplessness and hopelessness.* A considerable literature from cognitive clinical psychology has illuminated a number of strong predictive relationships between these overlapping variables and the onset of depression.

4. *Being female.* It is well established that depression is more frequently diagnosed in females than in males. Adolescent females may be particularly 'at risk' because of the

accumulation of stressors at a time of transition. Thus, where going through puberty, changing from primary to secondary school and family discord or break-up occur together, females may be especially at risk to develop depression.

5. *Living in poverty*. Epidemiological studies have identified poverty as an important risk factor for the development of depression. This may be because it is related to other risk factors such as more frequently experiencing stressors, having low self-esteem, poor self-efficacy and so on.

In light of our previous discussions concerning the possible 'culture boundness' of depression, let us acknowledge that the notion of 'depression', of biological and individual risk factors, reflects 'Western biological individualism'. However, being female and living in poverty suggest that contextual and environmental factors are also relevant to this North American idea of depression. It is therefore interesting to note that minority groups have been a target for intervention programmes specifically aimed at preventing depressive disorder.

North American estimates for the prevalence of clinical depression among the general population are generally between 9 and 14 per cent. However, of these, possibly only 20 per cent receive professional help. The situation for members of minority cultural groups may be even worse. For instance, epidemiological research in California has found that only 11 per cent of Mexican Americans who met diagnostic criteria for DSM (*Diagnostic and Statistical Manual* of the American Psychiatric Association) disorders had sought mental health services, compared with 22 per cent of similarly diagnosed non-Hispanic whites in the same catchment area. Such results suggest that minority groups may underutilize 'conventional' health services when it comes to mental disorder. If it is the case that minority groups underutilize treatment services, then greater emphasis might profitably be given to preventive interventions. An example of this would be Projecto Bienestar.

Projecto Bienestar targeted women who currently had no or only mild depressive symptoms, but who were nonetheless at high risk for developing depression of clinical severity. Emphasizing the importance of environmental resources, the project sought to strengthen individuals' capacities for coping with stressors. Two types of intervention were used. First, replicating the cultural norm of natural helpers (Servidoras) found in low-income communities of southern California, was a one-to-one intervention to assist the at-risk women. Second, there was a peer group intervention (Merienda educativa) which was organized and led by Servidoras. While the one-to-one intervention showed no positive effects in terms of preventing the onset of depression, the Merienda group intervention did. The effectiveness of the group intervention seems to have been accounted for by the benefits derived from it by women with relatively moderate depressive symptomatology, rather than those with relatively milder or relatively greater symptomatology. These results, while encouraging in terms of the potential efficacy of preventive intervention, also warn of the likely complexities involved in matching preventive interventions to risk factors, especially across a range of migrant cultures at risk of developing a 'foreign' disorder, such as depression (see Vega & Murphy, 1990, for further details).

## The interplay of risk factors

Coie and colleagues (1993), while supporting the risk factor approach, have also emphasized its complexities: there is no simple one-to-one relationship between a risk factor and a disorder. A particular risk factor—say, family discord—can be a risk factor for many different disorders. A particular disorder may also have many different risk factors, some of which may only occasionally be present. The salience of risk factors may also fluctuate developmentally. The idea of such 'sensitive periods' is that events occurring at one point in a person's life may have stronger effects on that person than the same event occurring at other times. The redundancy of a father may have different effects on his son depending on whether the son is 4 or 14. As a final point, the accumulation of risk factors is likely to increase vulnerability to disorder. The stressor which finally results in some form of breakdown may not be the most important stressor, but simply the one which stretched the person beyond his or her coping abilities. Where risk factors and stressors relate to social norms they are necessarily going to be a product of particular cultural beliefs. Risk factors may therefore show significant variation across cultures.

Schumaker (1996) illustrates this point by drawing our attention to the cultural assumptions which underlie theorizing about depressive thinking. Central to Beck's cognitive theory of depression is the idea that people who are depressed have a negative view of themselves. For example, they attribute their failure to cope with stressors to faults within themselves when there may be other explanations of their failure. This model fits well the individualistic orientation of North American society for which it was developed. Within this context, the attribution of negative events to personal shortcomings can be seen as a risk factor for developing depression. With increasing negative events exceeding a person's ability to cope—and that person increasingly attributing his or her failure to personal weaknesses—low self-esteem, self-depreciation, low mood and 'cognitive distortions' can worsen into a state of clinical depression. This way of thinking reflects the individual who has neither competed nor won, who is not trying to 'develop' himself or herself, and who is not a success. Arguably it is because 'Western' individualism encourages these ways of thinking that those who fail to make the grade are at risk of depression. It is difficult to emphasize the goodness of the successful individual without also emphasizing the badness of the unsuccessful individual.

Research on postpartum depression has implicated the role of self-depreciatory cognitions in the disorder and some have advocated the use of cognitive therapy as an intervention.

'Dysfunctional cognitions', characteristic of a mother with postpartum depression, might include 'I should always know how best to care for my baby' or 'I should always be available for my baby'. Such thoughts relate to the idea that women should be personally responsible for their children. The thinking patterns associated with feeling unable to fulfil such responsibilities may lead to depression. But how might women in cultures where the responsibility of child rearing is shared with other women react to stressful situations? The Kipsigis of Kenya are a culture in which there is no evidence of postpartum depression. In the Kipsigis, child care responsibilities are shared, especially following childbirth. In fact at childbirth the mother is 'pampered' to such an extent that she is almost completely free of child care responsibilities. In such a context it would make little sense for the mother to have negative self-directed cognitions concerning her inability to cope with her new child, or her lack of availability to the child.

The above example illustrates how individual cognitions reflect cultural norms and that different cultures may have different norms which operate through individuals as risk factors for (different or similar) disorders. Some cultures, particularly 'Western' cultures, have norms which promote individualism. Having a poor opinion of oneself (i.e. low self-esteem) is recognized as a hallmark symptom of the 'Western' experience of depression (MacLachlan, 1987). Thus promotion of individualism as a way of being in the world has its particular costs as well as its particular benefits, its particular risk factors for disorder and its particular intervention methods.

By and large the ethos of risk reduction and prevention of disorder has much to recommend it and is certainly deserving of further research. However, these issues may be addressed in a rather narrow context. First, while the idea of prevention is a conceptual advance on treatment models, it can be argued that prevention does not go far enough. Second, the interventions being described are effectively attempts at social change; they usually aspire to change the health-related behaviour of target individuals or groups. We now turn to these two important issues.

## BEYOND PREVENTION

Within the field of psychological disorder interest has traditionally focused on what goes wrong (psychopathology), the process by which things go wrong (pathogenesis) and how to fix what has gone wrong (psychotherapy). The idea of preventing things going wrong ('psycho-inoculation'), is still orientated towards what makes for misery. An alternative approach is to consider what makes for health, what goes right, rather than what goes wrong. If we can identify the factors responsible for psychological wellness, then it should be possible to reach beyond the idea of preventing or avoiding a negative experience of disorder, to actively promoting a positive state of health. We have already seen how different cultures understand disease and disorder and therefore we should not be surprised if understandings of how to be healthly also vary across cultures.

Cowen (1994) has described five key pathways to wellness. Some of them reflect the 'Western' emphasis on individualism while others are possibly relevant outside that context. The pathways to wellness are:

1. *Forming wholesome early attachments.* This pathway recognizes the long dependency period of human childhood and the need for children to form warm, loving and secure relationships with their primary care-givers. Such relationships allow for the development of a strong sense of self on which the infant can build throughout life. The opportunity to form such attachments may be restricted not only by the experience of adverse psychological environments, but also by the experience of harsh physical living conditions. Thus poor shelter, nutrition and sanitation may all affect early attachments between children and care-givers.

2. *Acquiring age-appropriate competencies.* These competencies relate to cognitive and interpersonal skills, some of which may develop from sound early attachment relationships. In many societies the main fora for the acquisition of age-appropriate competencies are home and school. Yet in other societies school is not freely available and collective community responsibility 'schools' the developing child, thus blurring the distinction between family and school. As noted before, the notion of adolescence is not universal. In some cultures children move from childhood to adulthood, which is a difficult concept for many 'Westerners', quite literally weaned on the idea of adolescence, to comprehend. Different cultures often have the belief that their way of classifying human experience is based on some fundamental truth. In reality, different cultures not only respond to the world in different ways, but they also make the world into different places to live in.

3. *Exposure to settings favouring wellness.* This pathway to wellness is very much to do with living in communities which foster the individual's development, both psychologically and physically. We have previously discussed the ways in which different cultures afford support to their members and the mechanisms which different cultures present for dealing with grievances, including how one expresses and responds to distress.

4. *Having a sense of control over one's fate.* This pathway essentially relates to empowering individuals so that they feel some sense of control over events in their life. It could also easily relate to empowering groups or communities. As we have seen, ethnic minority groups may often suffer from poor health partly because they are disempowered. Other disempowered groups might include the poor, the elderly, the homeless and the disabled. They are disempowered by virtue of the fact that they have a weaker voice in 'mainstream society' and are therefore afforded a disproportionately small amount of resources. Those who have a sense of control feel that they can influence things which matter to them. Thus having a sense of control is a salient

issue for wellness across cultures. It should, however, be recognized that trusting in the benevolence of a God may also give communities and individuals a sense of being in control. This may be the case even if they live in objectively unpredictable physical environments subject to earthquakes, drought or hurricanes.

5. *Coping effectively with stress.* This is the final pathway to wellness described by Cowen. Some people appear to respond well to stress in that it gives them an 'edge', they rise to the occasion and perform better than they might in less stressful circumstances. Others, at the slightest sign of stress, go to pieces. The concept of 'hardiness' refers to the extent to which an individual sees stressful situations as a positive challenge to his or her capabilities. Often this relates to the degree of control the individual is able to assert over the situation. However, once again these findings come from 'Western' psychology where the ability of the individual to rise above his or her circumstances is seen as praiseworthy. In some cultures, struggling against natural forces, or other people, might be seen as morally wrong. In other cultures the individual's ability to put his or her trust in a deity may be seen as praiseworthy. Yet again, elsewhere, the willingness of individuals to turn to the wider community might be the most valued response an individual makes. Thus not only do sources of stress differ across cultures but the way in which stress should be dealt with also differs.

Not surprisingly this list of what makes for wellness overlaps with what is important for the prevention of disorder. Wellness and health are, however, more than just the absence of disorder. As we noted in Chapter 1, the World Health Organization (1948) described health as 'a complete state of physical, mental and social well-being and not merely the absence of disease or infirmity'. A focus on wellness can be seen as a very positive approach to differing cultures in that it seeks to understand the social mechanisms which exist within a community to maintain stability, harmony and the well-being of its members. Cultural groups will offer different solutions to the problem of forming wholesome early attachments, to acquiring age-appropriate competencies and having a sense of control over one's own fate. In one culture individuals may achieve some sense of control over their fate through believing in a benevolent deity who can be pleased and who will grant favours contingent on the practise of certain religious ritual. Other cultures may achieve the same sense of being able to influence the future by promoting the idea of individual primacy, that 'nobody can be a victim without their own consent', that 'if you try hard enough you can achieve anything', that 'you've got to look after number one'. Although these are radically different belief systems, they may well solve the same problem equally well, and each may be valuable in promoting wellness within a particular context.

## The contemporary creation of disordered communities

In his Keynote Address at the 1995 World Federation for Mental Health, Professor Albee emphasized that self-esteem, social support and stress management are important in preventing disorder and promoting health. Minority cultural groups, immigrants and peoples in transition immediately come to mind as groups who have their self-esteem challenged, social support mechanisms undermined and abilities to effectively cope with stress severely compromised. However, one subcultural distinction which is rarely drawn is that between rural and urban dwellers within the same cultural group, in the same country.

Where this distinction is drawn it is usually with reference to remote rural communities in the 'less developed' countries. An enduring belief is that such people are psychologically better off, because it is the stress of living in modern urban industrial societies which is responsible for much psychological and physical disorder. Epidemiological attempts to explore the extent of disorder in rural versus urbanized areas have been plagued by methodological problems such as the intensity of screening, the determination of what (severity) constitutes a case of disorder and the language of emotional distress (how problems are presented). However, a recent study by Mumford and colleagues (1996) reported that people living in isolated Chitral mountain villages in Pakistan, far from reporting stress-free lives, had, in fact, higher rates of disorder than is found in most 'Western' societies. This was especially so for women, for those from lower socioeconomic groups and for the less literate.

In other countries too we must seriously question the assumption that psychological disorder is a 'disease of modern living'. Within Europe there are various factors in train which may lead to increased rates of disorder in rural communities. European agricultural policies may have many knock-on social effects in rural farming areas. A commonly understood consequence of present EU policy is that for farms to be economic they will have to increase in size and/or productivity. Increased mechanization, EU production quotas and the increasing cost of agricultural land (to name but a few factors) are likely to lead to the situation where fewer people are able to make a living off the land. What will happen to the farmers who sell up? The most likely outcome is that they will go to cities where they hope jobs are more plentiful. Apart from these transient farmers being placed under the stress of economic desperation and unemployment, their leaving of rural communities will further exacerbate the problem of rural depopulation.

Within Ireland the rate of rural depopulation is at its highest since the Great Famine of the 1840s. This depopulation, and the likely consequences of EU policies, may further compromise the integrity of many rural communities. Already post offices, police stations, schools and churches have closed in many rural areas, where shells of houses testify to a once more populous past. What are the likely social effects of such changes? Social support networks are being seriously under-mined, as the number of venues for casual contact dimin-ishes. Social contact with like-minded people may be seen as an empowering experience resulting in the maintenance of self-esteem through a self-belief in what one is doing. Farm-ing has become a more isolating enterprise with increasing technology replacing the need for human labour and there-fore human contact on a daily basis. It cannot be coincidental that the rate of suicide in young Irish farmers has trebled over the last 10 years. No doubt the effects of depopulation also impinge on the individual's perceived ability to cope with stressful situations as they arise. Such stress undoubt-edly relates to trying to avoid going out of business and the shame of having to sell off a family's inheritance, perhaps of many generations.

This situation and many like it throughout Europe and elsewhere, are examples of disordered communities in the making: communities which cannot effectively support their own members. Communities denuded of their structural and functional integrity. Most tragically, these disordered com-munities are often being legislated for, even unwittingly planned for. The idea of the 'country life' being the ideal and an escape from the rat race of urban living, is not supported in studies of psychological disorder in rural and urban settings. However, we may well find that the 'country life' of the future will become increasing stressful for those dependent on farm-ing for their livelihood and that the rates of psychological disorder and related problems, such as suicide, will be much greater than in inner city areas.

## Psychology promoting public health

While the role of psychology in community care has been recognized for some time, its contributions to health promo-tion, primary care and public health have only recently begun to make an impact. Here we need not think of psychology as a

profession, but rather psychology as an active part of the
professional life of most practitioners. Vinck (1994) has recently outlined how health psychologists can contribute to the
promotion of public health. Most of the points he has made
also generalize to other professions, though psychologists
may be particularly well placed to carry out some of the functions. Vinck's suggestions include the following:

- forming a coalition with particular communities and collab-
  orating with the community at every stage of their attempt
  to enhance their well-being;
- translating data from large-scale epidemiological studies in
  terms of everyday behaviour;
- monitoring behaviours in the population which are of particular interest (e.g. high risk or protective behaviours);
- translating data gathered from monitoring into objectives
  for action;
- establishing the determinants of relevant behaviours;
- describing relevant aspects of the community's structure
  and function (e.g. subgroups, communication channels,
  leaders, values, resistances, etc.);
- designing    and    executing    'multimodal    multilevel'
  interventions;
- designing and applying health education programmes;
- designing, executing and evaluating project work;
- mobilizing financial, social and political support for action.

These points may be particularly useful when applied in a
cross-cultural context. Yet, in a sense, what Vinck is arguing
for is that each community should be treated as if it were a
separate culture. Hopefully this is also an emerging theme to
the reader of this book: that communities cultivate different
ways of living depending on the resources available to them,
their geographical, social, political and economic context. No
two communities are the same and these differences are often
simply of a greater degree when we compare communities
across cultures. It is also apparent that, for instance, urban
and rural, military and civilian, religious and secular, rich and

poor communities all differ and all are constituted of differing combinations of the above variables.

An important debate within the health promotion field is whether interventions should be directed at the individual or the system and context within which individuals live. In fact, psychology is usually identified with intervention at the individual level because of its concern with what motivates individuals to engage in, or avoid, certain health-related behaviours. The ethos of focusing on 'lifestyles' and choice is probably embedded in the Euro-American value of individual freedom. However, in this book we have repeatedly noted the importance of looking beyond the individual to the context in which behaviours occur. In reality, the focus of health promotion should not be the individual or the context, but the relation between the individual and the context. In practice, most health promotion efforts work at both levels.

For example, take an advertisement which warns against the dangers of cigarette smoking by presenting an image of a cigarette in the form of a coffin. At what level is this advertisement intended to work? At the individual level, a person may be made aware of an association between smoking and death and this awareness may scare them, so that they reflect on their own smoking behaviour. While this mechanism is theoretically possible I suspect that it is not an important factor in discouraging people from smoking. At the contextual level the same advertisement may reinforce non-smokers' beliefs that smoking is bad for you. When a smoker enters the company of such people he or she may be given very negative feedback about their smoking, and particularly smoking in the company of non-smokers. Thus, while the advertisement may have made smoking a salient topic, it may be the social pressure from others which has the greatest impact on smoking behaviour. Such pressure may result in the changing of norms and customs to the extent of certain areas being determined 'smoke-free zones'. This is not to deny that efforts should be directed at promoting the effectiveness of health messages at the level of individuals or market segments (Mac-Lachlan *et al.*, 1997c). Health promotion interventions should be seen as working at both the individual and contextual level. Changing social contexts is the next issue we address.

## Health promotion as social change

Given that health behaviours occur in the much broader context of society it is often the case that attempts to change health-related behaviours are attempts at social change. Yet there are often good reasons why communities may resist attempts to change them and there are also different ways of producing the change process. Intervention programmes are all too often aimed at achieving dramatic changes, the process of which does not take into account, or build upon, the social structures which already exist in a community or culture. While it is tempting to produce sweeping changes quickly, such attempts at change are often unsustainable because they fail to ignite the social forces which can integrate them into the life of the community. An alternative approach, which we will now explore, is to seek incremental improvement by integrating small-scale changes into the sociocultural fabric of community life (MacLachlan, 1996b).

Within any community, traditional knowledge, attitudes, beliefs and behaviours reflect a degree of equilibrium between forces which promote change and those which inhibit it. Customs relating to health have evolved, sometimes over thousands of years, in order to serve the well-being of the community and its members. If certain beliefs or practices have existed for hundreds of years then it is probably because they offer acceptable solutions to problems in living. Seeking to change people's health behaviour may therefore have ramifications which reach far beyond the ken of the health practitioner. Health service interventions may challenge not only a way of thinking about health or specific health behaviours, but also a complete way of understanding how the world works and one's place in it. Lewin's (1952) Field Theory describes how a balance exists when forces for change (driving forces) are equal to forces against change (restraining forces). Changing this balance therefore requires either an increase in driving forces or a decrease in restraining forces. So, for instance, the situation of many immigrant minorities into 'Western' cities is that they encounter powerful driving forces (in the form of the dominant biomedical health care system) to change their ideas and practices regarding health. At the same time they may experience a weakening of the restraining forces (in the form of 'loosening' of the social context for traditional beliefs and practices). Unless this 'decoupling' of their familiar belief system is effectively resisted, or the transitional process is carefully negotiated (through a health system which is tolerant of pluralism), individuals may be catapulted into a nihilistic state where they cannot accept either approach to health. This may result in their rejection of any coherent system of beliefs or practices regarding their health and/or other important aspects of their life.

This calamitous outcome is not, however, inevitable. According to Field Theory, the first stage of (successful) change involves 'unfreezing', or dismantling existing patterns of behaviour. Among immigrant groups this process may occur simply because there is insufficient social support for their traditional ways of living. In the second stage, 'change', new patterns of behaviour are adopted, hopefully ones that are adaptive to managing the imbalance brought about by the increase in driving forces and/or decrease in restraining forces. The third and final stage, 're-freezing', occurs when people are able to integrate their newly acquired knowledge, attitudes, beliefs or practices into their previously existing repertoire. A crucial issue in this whole change process will be the magnitude of change required. The term 'required' is used here to suggest that, for instance, in the case of an immigrant group, their new environment will require some degree of adaptation if they are to function successfully. The smaller the change required then the more readily it can be assimilated into the existing repertoire of skills. There are great difficulties when the message from health practitioners is not only that 'The way you're treating your child's measles is wrong', but 'Your whole system of understanding health and illness is wrong'!

We have already considered the situation where people have migrated to a country where they are lacking sufficient social support for their customary way of dealing with life, illness and well-being. What of the situation where immigrants find a place in a large and well-established community with similar cultural origins and practices to their own? Here there is sufficient social support to maintain traditional customs, health beliefs and practices. If members of this community are presented with requests to make large changes to their way of life then their most likely recourse will be to reject the need for change. The strength of support to resist such change may well exist in their new community. More than this, rejecting 'mainstream' health care services may even be seen as an important way of establishing your credentials as a committed member of your new community. Your allegiance to traditional values and willingness to reject 'neo-colonial' ideas of health and well-being may well earn you a 'place' and status in your new community. Indeed such a strategy can be seen as a very sensible way of managing the transition, for it reduces the degree of change required of you in adapting to your new environment.

Whether the health practitioner is attempting to intervene in promoting the health of an individual from a marginalized minority culture group or from a well-established subculture, the magnitude of the change being suggested will be of paramount importance. The smaller the proposed change, the less upheaval and adaptation it will require. The problem with this rationale is that, to be realistic, sometimes the health practitioner will feel that it is not a small change that is required, but a big change. It may be that health practices which were thought to be adaptive at a certain time and/or in a given place, are not adaptive in the presenting context. It is suggested that where significant changes in health behaviours are

sought, these should be driven through a series of complementary incremental steps in the direction of the desired
change. This incremental improvement philosophy argues for
the integrating of new ideas and behaviours into an existing
repertoire, prior to the next increment in the change process.
However, here the change process is not directed by the
health practitioner as such, but by the ease with which the
community can integrate new ideas; that is, by the rate of the
unfreezing–change–refreezing process. The practitioner, once
having indicated an initial small change, is then reactive to the
community's rate of change. The fact that the practitioner is
not proactive does not reduce his or her potency, for he or she
remains the facilitator of the community's change process.

Incremental improvement is essentially a strategic approach
to community change, operationalized through a series of
small steps in the desired direction. However, it is also a
learning process for the practitioner because he or she may
not know either the best way forward, or the ultimate destina-
tion of the change process. Ultimately the way in which a
community negotiates the change process, through umpteen
unfreezing–change–refreezing cycles, is a journey into the unknown. For the health practitioner this uncertainty can be a
frustration; so can the slow pace of change. Nonetheless, these
may be acceptable costs of a process which can enhance the
community's ownership of positive changes in health behaviour. The notion of attempting to achieve modest incremental improvements has also recently been emphasized by
Leviton (1996) in her review of the ways in which psychology
can be integrated with public health.

## Incremental improvement through learning from the community

Social institutions offer vectors for promoting health. The
workplace is a context in which a community atmosphere can
be utilized to enhance interventions. Community groups,

social clubs and schools are also alternative modes of intervention. Let us briefly consider a health promotion project
which used the community school as the site for intervention.
In the initial stage of this intervention we set out to learn from
the community, before trying to 'teach' to it (MacLachlan *et
al.*, 1997b). While this research took place in a Malawian government secondary school, the general principles of the intervention would probably be applicable in many schools, in
many countries. The focus of the intervention was to explore
and, where appropriate, to change unhealthy, knowledge, attitudes, beliefs and practices relating to HIV/AIDS.

The project, which extended over three years, began with a
qualitative search for existing ideas about HIV/AIDS. This
search included published written sources of information
such as newspaper reports, short stories, official government
statistics and press releases. The search also considered feedback from trainee teachers and their pupils, on lessons concerned with HIV/AIDS. Our search put particular emphasis
on the short story medium of communication, which is very
popular in Malawian newspapers. While this source would be
ignored by many conventional methods of research, we felt it
was an important aspect of cultural learning for secondary
school students. Many of the stories were clearly prescriptive
and moralistic. Whether one agrees with the prescription or
morals is not the point; what is important is to recognize that
this medium was feeding potentially influential messages into
the school community. Having identified these local understandings of HIV/AIDS and related sexual behaviour, we
checked them out with a panel of local 'experts' (lecturers,
medical practitioners, counsellors working with AIDS sufferers) asking them to add other important points which we
may have missed. Consequently, by removing and adding
items through several iterations, we derived 40 statements
covering HIV/AIDS and sexually related behaviour.

These statements covered a variety of themes including the
presentation of the disease (e.g. 'Everyone who loses a lot of

weight in a short time has AIDS', 'Some people who get AIDS become mentally disturbed', 'All babies of mothers infected with HIV are born with HIV'), its transmission (e.g. 'You can get AIDS from a mosquito if it bites you shortly after biting an AIDS victim', 'You can get AIDS from hugging', 'You can get AIDS from sharing a cup·with an AIDS victim'), folklore (e.g. 'Ministers of religion cannot get AIDS', 'A women cannot get HIV/AIDS if she has sex only once with an infected man', 'You cannot get AIDS if you have sex standing up') and treatment ('At present there is no cure for AIDS', 'AIDS victims can benefit from counselling'). Other items referred to methods of prevention and protection, sex education and statistics on AIDS/HIV (see MacLachlan *et al.*, 1997b). The pupils were required to give 'Yes' or 'No' answers to each of these statements. However, we were keen that this should not happen in a didactic teacher-to-pupil manner. We wanted to create a learning environment where pupils were actively involved in the learning process and, ideally, where they could learn from each other.

We achieved this active mutual learning by presenting the information in the format of a board game—based on Snakes and Ladders—which pupils played in groups of four to six with a facilitator (in this case a university student). Over four weekly sessions of playing the board game the percentage of correct responses significantly increased. This mode of intervention and our emphasis on the qualitative collation of local information are described as a modest example of how a community intervention to promote health can be undertaken. The importance of first learning from the community is underlined by some of the statements which were identified for the board game—statements which we certainly could not have foreseen as being an aspect of the pupil's understanding of AIDS and sexually related behaviour. Furthermore, while some health beliefs can be similarly constructed in different cultures (for instance, coping strategies, see Ager & MacLachlan, 1997), the relevance of others may differ substantially across cultures (for instance, health locus of control, see MacLachlan *et al.*, 1997a).

Identifying exactly what people think prior to a health promotion intervention is possibly the most important stage of the whole intervention process. It is the bedrock on which further ideas and behaviours must take root.

## THE BENEFITS OF COMMUNITY HEALTH PROMOTION PROGRAMMES

There have now been a number of large-scale health promotion programmes which focus on the community as the mechanism of intervention. The outcomes of these projects have generally been quite impressive and recent Japanese research suggests that investing financial resources in health promotion subsequently reduces the demand for (and cost of) medical care (Nakanishi *et al.*, 1996). One of the first major health promotion projects was the North Karelia Project, conducted in northern Finland, which focused on reducing the unusually high incidence of death from cardiovascular diseases in Finland. The interventions were focused on schools (e.g. healthy heart lifestyle programmes), community centres (e.g. low-fat cooking classes), work sites (e.g. smoking cessation courses) and so on. A five-year follow-up study compared the citizens of Karelia State with a neighbouring state which did not experience the intensive health promotion intervention. The risk of cardiovascular diseases decreased by 17 per cent in men and 11 per cent in women and these improvements were maintained over a 10-year follow-up. The North Karelia Project, initiated in 1973, thus demonstrated that community interventions could be effective in combating serious diseases and so reducing mortality.

Another ground-breaking community health promotion initiative was the Stanford Three-Community Study which was undertaken by Stanford University in three small communities in northern California. The primary aim of the project was to assess the influence of a mass media programme on, once again, cardiovascular diseases. Two of the communities received the same mass media programme which included television, radio, mailing of information sheets, newspaper reports and stories and billboards. In addition, one of these communities also received an intervention programme (including smoking cessation, weight loss, diet enhancement and physical exercise) which was targeted at high-risk persons, identified by questionnaire assessment. The third community received only the initial risk assessment and neither the media programme nor the behavioural intervention programme. The risk of cardiovascular diseases significantly decreased in the first two communities, but not the third. In the community which received the additional behavioural intervention, the rate of decrease was greater, but over time each community achieved a reduction in risk for cardiovascular disease of between 25 and 30 per cent. The significance of the Stanford Three-Community Study is that it demonstrated that health promotion programmes could be targeted at relatively small communities and that the improvement in health could be community-wide rather than restricted to a few high-risk individuals.

Many other community-based health promotion programmes are now underway in different parts of the world and this seems to be a mode of intervention which is increasingly recognized as valuable. However, probably the majority of such programmes target a geographical community without taking into account the different cultural groups which may constitute the geographical community. As such, the means of health promotion employed may favour certain sections of the community over members of minority groups. It is therefore important to consider what these factors might be and to think through health promotion techniques which can be sensitive to the needs of different cultures.

Douglas (1995) has described the importance of developing 'anti-racist health promotion strategies'. Writing about the development of health promotion in Britain, she identifies three phases of racist social policies since the early 1960s. The assimilation phase was characterized by health promotion information being given to cultural minorities to encourage them to conform to British lifestyle norms. This was actioned through a proliferation of health promotion literature on family planning, the diets of Asian families and tuberculosis. An implicit goal of this phase was the modification of 'deviant' cultural minority lifestyles in order to allow for assimilation into the British way of life.

The next phase was one of social integration where minority groups need not completely abandon their cultural heritage. Thus in the late 1960s a greater sense of tolerance was emerging towards differences between mainstream British society and minority groups within it. A greater emphasis was put on physical and cultural differences, an example of this being the increased interest in hereditary conditions such as sickle-cell anaemia. However, this sort of 'tolerance' reflected a move away from integration. The 1970s and 1980s were associated with a concern to compare the behaviour of individuals from one culture with that of individuals from another (usually mainstream British) culture. Much of the research at this time reflected a medical model concerned with how illness and disease (such as tuberculosis, rickets, mental illness, perinatal mortality and low birth weight) affected minority cultural groups.

The model of health promotion based on this third phase attempted to 'educate' individuals to adopt more 'appropriate' lifestyles. As such, it could be seen as targeted at 'deficit behaviours', where the lifestyle or the culture was 'blamed' for the individual's poor health. An often-quoted example of this is the Rickets Campaign of the early 1980s which was the first health education campaign specifically targeted towards minority culture communities. As we have previously discussed, a poor diet, particularly one lacking in vitamin D, and the custom of covering almost all of the body, thereby preventing exposure to sunlight, have been implicated in the cause of rickets in Britain. The Rickets Campaign therefore emphasized the importance of the Asian community changing its diet in order to have a higher intake of vitamin D. Critics have pointed out that there was quite a different emphasis in combating rickets in the British (mainly white) population during the Second World War, where the problem was addressed through the supplementing of particular foods with vitamin D (e.g. margarine). This later strategy reflected the assumption that rickets was caused in the British population by poverty, yet 40 years later it was seen as being caused in Asians by cultural styles of living, including diet.

Douglas's critique of British health promotion and social policy emphasizes that illness among minority cultural groups is often attributed to their alternative cultural practices rather than to the relative poverty in which many minority communities live. She also stresses that the illness targets for health promotion interventions are often those of concern to (predominantly white) health professionals, rather than members of the minority culture groups themselves. Douglas's main point appears to be that the position which minority cultures are 'put in' by mainstream society should be a major interest of health promoters and more generally of social policy (see also Ahmad, 1996). Thus experiences of poverty, broader aspects of socioeconomic position, racial discrimination and so on, should be recognized. These are indeed important points but, at the same time, there is also a risk of placing too much emphasis on the broader sociopolitical and economic context and subtracting from the value of a cultural level analysis.

It is clear that some cultures engage in behaviours detrimental to their health, despite being relatively 'comfortable' on a broad range of social, economic and political indicators. One comparison might be between the Islanders of the Western Hebrides of Scotland and the inhabitants of the Norfolk Broads of England. The exceptionally high rates of alcoholism in the former group could be attributed to some aspects of social disadvantage. It would generally not be attributed to aspects of Hebridean Islander's relative advantage. However, the difference might more appropriately be attributed to the different heritage of Celtic and Anglo-Saxon peoples and to the particular ways in which these two cultures encourage socializing.

A major concern with regard to promoting health in different cultures should be to avoid not only 'blaming the victim' of disadvantage but also to avoid the well-known psychological actor–observer effect. In the present context this is demonstrated by illness being observed in a particular cultural community and the 'observers' (those looking on, in this case 'mainstream society') attributing its cause to the behaviour of the minority cultural group—the actors. At the same time, the actors (those immediately experiencing the problems) attribute the cause of it to the context in which they are acting out their lives. The focus of the actors and observers is on each other as the cause of the problem. Racism is usually thought of as coming from the observer and being directed at the hapless actors. Yet by this formulation it could also come from the actors and be directed towards the hapless observers. My point is therefore that the context and the culture interact in complex ways to define how any group of people lives.

Changes in social, economic, geographical or political contexts may also require cultures to change if the culture is going to remain an adaptive medium through which its members can live in the world. The situation in relation to all cultures and their broader context is therefore complex (involving many interrelated variables) and dynamic (in a process of continual change for the purpose of adaptation). It would indeed be a fallacy to believe that some cultural practices are not maladaptive in certain contexts. Anyone who doubts this need only observe the after-effects of the first day's sun bathing by English tourists on the Spanish Costa del Sol— ouch! On a more serious note, the high incidence of skin cancer among white Australians may be a result of the failure of their cultural practices to adapt to their present environment. It could be argued that health promotion directed at getting white people to cover up, spend less time in the sun, wear protective creams and so on, is directed at 'deficit' behaviour. However, this 'deficit', as with the case of vitamin D and rickets among British Asians, should not be seen as intrinsic to a particular cultural group *per se*, but particular to certain behaviours in certain contexts which may put one cultural group at greater risk than another.

The benchmark of culturally sensitive, but not racist, health promotion must be the treatment of different cultural groups with the same integrity and respect. There can be nothing racist in recognizing that different groups of people, living in the world in different ways, may have different needs for maintaining their health. However, such a recognition must in no way distract our attention from the health consequences of living in poverty and experiencing racial discrimination. It is a travesty that, in many of the world's so-called 'developed' countries, minority cultures are treated opportunistically as cheap labour and do not have the same social welfare rights as the majority of citizens. What sort of host culture allows such a situation to persist? This is as much a moral question as it is a psychological, sociopolitical or economic one. It is, nonetheless, a question which we should all address in our efforts to promote health within all cultures.

## GUIDELINES FOR PROFESSIONAL PRACTICE

1. The dramatic increase in the health of citizens of most industrialized countries can be attributed to improvements in public health, such as safe drinking water, efficient sewage systems and better nutrition, rather than to biotechnological innovations in treatment. Clinicians should be proactive in identifying the ways in which health can be promoted, rather than being solely concerned with reactively treating problems as they arise.

2. The relatively poor health of many minority cultural groups may be attributed to their more limited access to health-promoting initiatives, rather than to a relatively higher incidence of disease or disorder. With equal access to health-promoting initiatives and with the provision of similarly health promoting environments, the health of minority cultural groups can be equal to the health of majority cultural groups. However, clinicians may need to work with different mediums for promoting health in different cultural groups.

3. Relatively simple behaviours (e.g. eating breakfast daily, moderate use of alcohol, sleeping seven to eight hours daily) have been shown to be significantly associated with longer life span. It would therefore seem that certain behaviours are strongly health promoting, while others are strongly health threatening (e.g. physical inactivity, smoking cigarettes, eating between meals). Clinicians should not, however, assume that the same 'package' of health-promoting or health-demoting behaviours will have identical effects across cultural groups. Presumably the effects of some of these behaviours depend on what else you do, and there may be some cultural practices which are especially effective or defective in promoting health. This is an empirical issue.

4. While cultural sensitivity (awareness of cultural issues) is important for clinicians, it is not sufficient. Clinicians must also be culturally competent and this requires personal experience of working with different cultural groups. This book is intended to enhance cultural sensitivity and to encourage clinicians to strive towards cultural competence.

5. Although health promotion has historically focused on physical health, its value in mental health is now well recognized. A recent US report has highlighted 10 issues to be considered when clinicians are working with different cultural groups and seeking to prevent mental disorders. These points in themselves constitute guidelines and may be used to help individual clinicians,

or clinical teams, review their interventions across cultures.

6. Specific risk factors can be identified for particular disorders. Sometimes these risk factors may be particularly prominent in a cultural group. For instance, experiencing a severe stressor, having low self-esteem and living in poverty have been identified as risk factors for depression. Recent immigrants often experience stress as a result of their transition. They may find that the minority cultural group of which they are a member is discriminated against, with the result that many of them feel undervalued and have low self-esteem. Furthermore, immigrant groups are often economically disadvantaged such that they will be living in poor housing and possibly without employment or full access to social services. In such cases whole communities may be at risk for developing depression. Thus minority cultural groups may deserve special efforts to be made in preventing disorder and promoting health.

7. Culture influences the way in which people think. Many 'Western' cultures emphasize the primacy of the individual and of the individual achieving success. Such an emphasis may predispose people in these cultures to negatively react to the realization that they are not, in fact, the outstanding individuals that they (and their friends) would like them to be. A loss of belief in the self is a central 'symptom' of depression. Thus 'Western' cultures may be seen to predispose to this experience of depression. Cultures emphasizing other values may predispose to different reactions. In some sense, then, culture itself can be thought of as a risk factor.

8. Clinicians should analyse different cultures in an attempt to identify how each seeks to solve certain common problems: how to deal with stress, how to acquire age-appropriate competencies, or how to form wholesome early attachments. These pathways to health are the routes which clinicians must work through even though they may be foreign to the clinician.

9. A widespread assumption is that life in urban communities is more stressful than life in rural communities. Recent research does not support this belief. Furthermore, the urbanization of many societies may result in rural life becoming more stressful through, for instance, the reduction in available social support networks. Contemporary government and international policies may place people in rural and urban areas at greater risk for developing disorders. The health implications of such policies deserve the attention of clinicians who wish to facilitate health promotion.

10. Health promotion will often require clinicians to work with communities, not as leaders but as facilitators of social change. In this role clinicians can be catalysts for better health by empowering people to take charge of their well-being. This role may involve monitoring behaviour, translating data, mobilizing resources, and so on, rather than being seen as the agent of change.

11. Incremental improvements to health is a philosophy of change where the magnitude of change which occurs at any given time is determined by factors within the community the clinician is seeking to serve, rather than by the aspirations of the clinician. Often it will require the clinician to be prepared to learn from the community before attempting to assist it.

12. There is now strong evidence that community health promotion programmes can be effective in reducing serious diseases and mortality, that health gains need not be restricted to high-risk individuals but can be community-wide and that they can be specifically targeted to minority cultural groups. It is important that we learn from past mistakes and do not see minority cultural lifestyles as deviant or deficient. However, it is equally important not to cocoon minority or majority cultural behaviours in 'cultural relativism'. It is reasonable to assume that some behaviours relate more strongly to health than to disorder, and it is the clinician's responsibility to identify and advise on these, treating each cultural group differently, but with equal respect.

# POSTSCRIPT

*May you live in interesting times* (Chinese proverb)

In times now past the study of different cultures was the exotica of social sciences. Incomprehension of another culture was taken as confirmation of the legitimacy of ethnocentric world views. Now the study of culture is an imperative for human existence. In evolutionary terms we have been catapulted into a multicultural hot-house. We kick and struggle with each other and occasionally, and too frequently, betray our universal virtues with murderous rampages through humanity. These rampages often have an explicit cultural or racial element and where they may not, then these are often grafted on. It is everyday experience that multiculturalism is a big problem for a small planet.

This book has set out a path through the complexity of culture and health. Culture affects health even for those unaware of their cultural heritage and unconcerned about their health. It is an inescapable interplay even when you resist being a player. Many clinicians resist being players. They stand behind the glass of scientific objectivity which 'objectifies' the patient. Patients (or clients) ought not to be the 'object' of our activity but the *subject* of our concern, and we must be concerned with how their experience of the world contributes to the problems which they present.

Some of the themes emphasized in this book have included: the dynamic tension between keeping the individual foreground and cultural background in perspective; considering the social, economic and political context in which different cultural groups operate; seeing the communities which people live in, especially immigrant groups, as resources for promoting health; recognizing the wholeness of health and illness rather than splitting it into mind and body and developing tolerance for pluralistic approaches to health. The guidelines at the end of each chapter have tried to give practical suggestions for action. Only through such action can you set out on your own path through this most perplexing and fascinating forest of human health and culture.

# REFERENCES

Ager, A. & MacLachlan, M. (1997) Measuring coping strategies in Malawian students. *Psychology and Health* (in press).

Ahdieh, L. & Hahn, R.A. (1996) Use of terms 'Race', 'Ethnicity' and 'National Origin': a review of articles in the American Journal of Public Health, 1980–89. *Ethnicity and Health*, **1**(1), 95–98.

Ahmad, W.I.U. (Ed.) (1996) *'Race' and Health in Contemporary Britain*. Buckingham: Open University Press.

Airhihenbuwa, C.O. (1995) *Health and Culture: Beyond the Western Paradigm*. Thousand Oaks, CA: Sage.

Alarcon, R.D. & Foulks, E.F. (1995) Personality disorders and culture: contemporary clinical views (A). *Cultural Diversity and Mental Health*, **1**(1), 3–17.

Allen, T. (1992) Taking culture seriously. In T. Allen and A. Thomas (Eds) *Poverty and Development in the 1990s*. Oxford: Oxford University Press.

Anderson, E.A. (1987) Preoperative preparation for cardiac surgery facilitates recovery, reduces psychological distress, and reduces the incidence of acute postoperative hypertension. *Journal of Consulting and Clinical Psychology*, **55**, 513–520.

Antonovsky, A. (1987) *Unraveling the Mystery of Health: How People Manage Stress and Stay Well*. San Francisco: Jossey-Bass.

Asano, S. (1994) Unrelated bone marrow donor registry in Japan. *Bone Marrow Transplantation*, **13**, 699–700.

Baider, L., Kaufman, B., Ever-Hadani, P. & De-Nour, A.K. (1996) Coping with additional stresses: comparative study of healthy and cancer patient new immigrants. *Social Science and Medicine*, **42**(7), 1077–1084.

Baumeister, R.F. (1991) *Meanings of Life*. New York: Guilford Press.

Belloc, N.B. & Breslow, L. (1972) Relationship of physical health status and health practices. *Preventive Medicine*, **5**, 409–421.

Bernal, M.A. & Castro, F.G. (1994) Are clinical psychologists prepared for service and research with ethnic minorities? Report of a decade of progress. *American Psychologist*, **49**(9), 707–805.

Berry, J.W. & Kim, U. (1988) Acculturation and mental health. In P. Dasen, J.W. Berry and N. Sartorius (Eds) *Health and Cross-Cultural Psychology*. London: Sage.

Berry, J.W. (1990) Psychology of acculturation: understanding individuals moving between cultures. In R.W. Brislin (Ed.) *Applied Cross-Cultural Psychology*. Newbury Park: Sage.

Berry, J.W. (1994) Cross-cultural health psychology. Paper presented at International Congress of Applied Psychology, Madrid, 17–22 July.

Bishop, G. (1996) East meets West: illness, cognition and behaviour in Singapore. Paper presented at the 10th European Health Psychology Society Conference, Dublin, 4–6 September.

Black, J. (1989) *Child Health in a Multicultural Society*. London: British Medical Journal Publications.

Bochner, S. (1982) The social psychology of cross-cultural relations. In S. Bochner (Ed.) *Cultures in Contact: Studies in Cross-Cultural Interaction*. Oxford: Pergamon Press.

Bond, M.H. (1991) Chinese values and health: a cultural-level examination. *Psychology and Health*, **5**, 137–152.

Bond, M.H. (1988) Finding universal dimensions of individual variation in multicultural studies of values: the Rokeach and Chinese values survey. *Journal of Personality and Social Psychology*, **55**, 1009–1015.

Boyd, J.H. & Weissman, M.M. (1981) Epidemiology of affective disorder. *Archives of General Psychiatry*, **38**, 1039–1046.

Brady, M. (1995) Culture in treatment, culture as treatment: a critical appraisal of developments in addiction programmes for indigenous North Americans and Australians. *Social Science and Medicine*, **41**, 1487–1498.

Branscombe, N.R. & Wann, D.L. (1992) Role of identification with a group, arousal, categorization process, and self-esteem in sports spectator aggression. *Human Relations*, **45**, 1013–1033.

Breslow, L. & Enstrom, J.E. (1980) Persistence of health habits and their relationship to mortality. *Preventive Medicine*, **9**, 469–483.

Brislin, R., Cushner, K., Cherrie, C. & Yong, M. (1986) *Intercultural Interactions: A Practical Guide*. Newbury Park, C.A.: Sage.

Brown, G. & Harris, T. (1978) *The Social Origins of Depression*. London: Tavistock Publications.

Brown, C.M. & Segal, R. (1996) The effects of health and treatment perceptions on the use of prescribed medication and home re-

medies among African American and white American hyperten-
sives. *Social Science and Medicine*, **43**, 903–917.

Carr, S.C., Watters, P.A. & MacLachlan, M. (1996) Beyond cognitive
tolerance: towards the edge of chaos. Paper presented at the European Health Psychology Society Conference, Dublin, 4–6
September.

Casimir, G.J. & Morrison, B.J. (1993) Rethinking work with 'multicultural populations'. *Community Mental Health Journal*, **29**(6),
547–559.

Cheng, S.T. (1994) A critical review of the Chinese Koro. Paper
presented at International Congress of Applied Psychology,
Madrid, 17–22 July.

Chirimuuta, R. & Chirimuuta, R. (1989) *AIDS, Africa and Racism.*
London: Free Association Books.

Clark, M., cited in R.C. Simons & C.C. Hughes (Eds) (1985) *The
Culture Bound Syndromes: Folk Illnesses of Psychiatric and Anthropological Interest*. Dordrecht: D. Reidel.

Coie, J.D., Watt, N.F., West, S.G. *et al.* (1993) The science of prevention: a conceptual framework and some directions for a national
research program. *American Psychologist*, **48**(10), 1013–1022.

Collett, P. (1982) Meetings and misunderstandings. In S. Bochner
(Ed.) *Cultures in Contact: Studies in Cross-Cultural Interaction*. Oxford: Pergamon Press.

Cowen, E. (1994) The enhancement of psychological wellness: challenges and opportunities. *American Journal of Community Psychology*, **22** (2), 149–179.

DeSantis, L. & Halberstein, R. (1992) The effects of immigration on
the health care system of south Florida. *Human Organization*,
**51**(3), 223–234.

Dollard, J. (1935) *Criteria for the Life History: With Analysis of Six
Notable Documents*. New Haven: Yale University Press.

Dona, G. & Berry, J.W. (1994) Acculturation attitudes and acculturative stress of Central American refugees. *International Journal of
Psychology*, **29**(1), 57–70.

Douglas, J. (1995) Developing anti-racist health promotion strategies. In R. Bunton, S. Nettleton & R. Burrows (Eds) *The Sociology
of Health Promotion: Critical Analyses of Consumption, Lifestyle and
Risk*. London: Routledge, pp. 70–77.

Draguns, J. (1990) Applications of cross-cultural psychology in the
field of mental health. In R.W. Brislin (Ed.) *Applied Cross-Cultural
Psychology*. Newbury Park: Sage.

Eisenbruch, M. (1990) Classification of natural and supernatural
causes of mental distress: development of a mental distress ex-

planatory model questionnaire. *Journal of Nervous and Mental Disease*, **178**(11), 712–719.

Festinger, L.A. (1957) *A Theory of Cognitive Dissonance*. Stanford: Stanford University Press.

Fish, J.M. (1995) Why psychologists should learn some anthropology. *American Psychologist*, **50**, 44–45.

Flanagan, J.C. (1954) The critical incident technique. *Psychological Bulletin*, **51**, 327–358.

Garcia-Campayo, J., Campos, R., Marcos, G *et al.* (1996) Somatisation in primary care in Spain II: Differences between somatisers and psychologisers. *British Journal of Psychiatry*, **168**, 348–353.

Garfinkel, H. (1967) *Studies in Ethnomethodology*. Cambridge: Polity Press.

Garner, D.M. & Garfinkle, P.E. (1980) Sociocultural factors in the development of anorexia nervosa. *Psychological Medicine*, **10**, 647–656.

Geertz, H. (1968) Latah in Java: A theoretical paradox. *Indonesia*, **3**, 93–104.

Gordon, T., Garcia-Palmieri, M.R., Kagan, A., Kannel, W.B. & Schiffman, J. (1974) Differences in coronary heart disease in Famingham, Honolulu and Puerto Rico. *Journal of Chronic Disease*, **27**, 329–344.

Halpern, D. (1993) Minorities and mental health. *Social Science and Medicine*, **36**(5), 597–607.

Hancock, T. & Perkins, F. (1985) The Mandala of Health: a conceptual model and teaching tool. *Health Promotion*, **24**, 8–10.

Harris, M. (1980) *Cultural Materialism: The Struggle for a Science of Culture*. New York: Vintage Books.

Haviland, W.A. (1983) *Human Evolution and Prehistory* (2nd edn). New York: CBS College Publishing.

Heller, C. & Monahan, A. (1977) cited in Winnett *et al.* (1989)

Ho, D.Y.F. (1985) Cultural values and professional issues in clinical psychology: implications from the Hong Kong experience. *American Psychologist*, **40** (11), 1212–1218.

Hofstede, G. (1991) *Cultures and Organizations*. London: HarperCollins Publishers.

Hofstede, G. (1980) *Culture's Consequences: International differences in work-related values*. Beverly Hills, CA: Sage.

Hofstede, G. (1986) Cultural differences in teaching and learning. *International Journal of Intercultural Relations*, **10**, 301–320.

Hughes, C.C. (1985) Culture-bound or construct-bound? The syndromes and DSM-III. In R.C. Simons & C.C. Hughes (Eds) *The*

*Culture Bound Syndromes: Folk Illnesses of Psychiatric and Anthropological Interest*. Dordrecht: D. Reidel, pp. 3–24.

Ilechukwu, S.T.C. (1989) Approaches to psychotherapy in Africans: do they have to be non-medical? *Culture, Medicine and Psychiatry*, **13**, 419–435.

Ilola, L.M. (1990) Culture and health. In R.W. Brislin (Ed.) *Applied Cross-Cultural Psychology*. Newbury Park: Sage.

Inkeles, A. (1969) Making men modern: on the causes and consequences of individual change in six developing countries. *American Journal of Comparative Sociology*, **75**, 208–225.

Jenkins, C.N.H., Le, T., McPhee, S.J., Stewart, S. & Ha, N.T. (1996) Health care access and prevention care among Vietnamese immigrants: do traditional beliefs and practices pose barriers? *Social Science and Medicine*, **43**, 1049–1056.

Jilek, W.G. & Jilek-Aall, L.M. (1984) Intercultural psychotherapy: experiences from North American Indian patients. *Curare*, **7**, 161–166.

Kanyangale, M. & MacLachlan, M. (1995) Critical incidents for refugee counsellors: an investigation of indigenous human resources. *Counselling Psychology Quarterly*, **8**(1), 89–101.

Kareem, J. (1992) The Nafsiyat Intercultural Therapy Centre: ideas and experience in intercultural therapy. In J. Kareem and R. Littlewood (Eds) *Intercultural Therapy: Themes, Interpretations and Practice*. Oxford: Blackwell Scientific Publications.

Kareem, J. & Littlewood, R. (Eds) (1992) *Intercultural Therapy: Themes, Interpretations and Practice*. Oxford: Blackwell Scientific Publications.

Kenny, M.G. (1985) Paradox lost: the latah problem revisited. In R.C. Simons & C.C. Hughes (Eds) *The Culture-Bound Syndromes: Folk Illnesses of Psychiatric and Anthropological Interest*. Dordrecht: D. Reidel, pp. 63–76.

Khandelwal, S.K., Sharan, P. & Saxena, S. (1995) Eating disorders: an Indian perspective. *International Journal of Social Psychiatry*, **41**(2), 132–146.

Kleinman, A. (1980) *Patients and Healers in the Context of Culture*. Berkeley: University of California Press.

Kluckhohn, C. & Kroeber, A. (1952) Culture. *Peabody Museum Papers* (Harvard University), **67**(1).

Knight, T. (1994) Personal communication, Department of Classics, University of Malawi.

Kobasa, S.C.O., Maddi, S.R., Puccetti, M.C. & Zola, M.A. (1985) Effectiveness of hardiness, exercise and social support as resources against illness. *Journal of Psychosomatic Research*, **29**, 525–533.

Lago, C. & Thompson, J. (1996) *Race, Culture and Counselling*. Buckingham: Open University Press.

Landrine, H. & Klonoff, E.A. (1992) Culture and health-related schemas: a review and proposal for interdisciplinary integration. *Health Psychology*, **11**(4), 267–276.

Levine, R.V. & Bartlett, K. (1984) Pace of life, punctuality, and coronary heart disease in six countries. *Journal of Cross-Cultural Psychology*, **15**(2), 233–255.

Leviton, L. (1996) Integrating psychology and public health: challenges and opportunities. *American Psychologist*, **51**(1), 42–51.

Lewin, K. (1952) Group decision and social change. In T. Newcomb and E. Hartley (Eds) *Readings in Social Psychology*. New York: Holt, Rinehart & Winston, (pp. 459–473).

Liang, R., Chiu, E., Chan, T.K. & Hawkins, B. (1994) An unrelated marrow donor registry in Hong Kong. *Bone Marrow Transplantation*, **13**, 697–698.

Lipton, J.A. & Marbach, J.J. (1984) Ethnicity and the pain experience. *Social Science and Medicine*, **19**(12), 1279–1298.

Littlewood, R. (1992b) How universal is something we can call therapy? In J. Kareem & R. Littlewood (Eds) *Intercultural Therapy: Themes, Interpretations and Practice*. Oxford: Blackwell Scientific Publications.

Littlewood, R. (1992a) Towards an intercultural therapy. In J. Kareem & R. Littlewood (Eds) *Intercultural Therapy: Themes, Interpretations and Practice*. Oxford: Blackwell Scientific Publications.

Lobo, A., Garcia-Campayo, J., Campos, R. *et al.* (1996) Somatisation in primary care in Spain, I: Estimates of prevalence and clinical characteristics. *British Journal of Psychiatry*, **168**, 344–353.

MacLachlan, M. (1987) Self-esteem in affective disorder. In H. Dent (Ed.) *Clinical Psychology: Research and Developments*. London: Croom Helm.

MacLachlan, M. (1996a) From sustainable change to incremental improvement: the psychology of community rehabilitation. In S.C. Carr & J.F. Schumaker (Eds) *Psychology and the Developing World*. Westport, C.T.: Greenwood Publishing Group.

MacLachlan, M. (1996b) Identifying problems in community health promotion: an illustration of the nominal group technique in AIDS education. *Journal of the Royal Society of Health*, **116**(3), 143–148.

MacLachlan, M., Ager, A. & Brown, J. (1997a) Health locus of control in Malawi: a failure to support the cross-cultural validity of the HLOCQ. *Psychology and Health*, **12**, 33–38.

MacLachlan, M. & Carr, S.C. (1994a) From dissonance to tolerance: towards managing health in tropical cultures. *Psychology and Developing Societies*, **6**(2), 119–129.

MacLachlan, M. & Carr, S.C. (1994b) Managing the AIDS crisis in Africa: in support of pluralism. *Journal of Management in Medicine*, **8**(4), 45–53.

MacLachlan, M., Chimombo, M. & Mpemba, N. (1997b) AIDS education for youth through active learning: a school-based approach from Malawi. *International Journal of Educational Development*, **17**(1), 41–50.

MacLachlan, M., Connacher, A.A. & Jung, R.T. (1991) Psychological aspects of dietary weight loss and medication with the atypical beta agonist BRL 26830A in obese subjects. *International Journal of Obesity*, **15**, 27–35.

MacLachlan, M., Nyando, M.C. & Nyirenda, T. (1995) Attributions for admission to Zomba Mental Hospital: implications for the development of mental health services in Malawi. *International Journal of Social Psychiatry*, **41**(2), 79–87.

MacLachlan, M., Carr, S.C., Fardell, S., Maffesoni, G. & Cunningham, J. (1997c) Transactional analysis of communication styles in HIV/AIDS advertisements. *Journal of Health Psychology* **2**(1), 67–74.

MacLachlan, M. & McAuliffe, E. (1993) Critical incidents for psychology students in a refugee camp: implications for counselling. *Counselling Psychology Quarterly*, **6**(1), 3–11.

Magnusson, A. & Axelsson, J. (1993) The prevalence of seasonal affective disorder is low among descendants of Icelandic emigrants in Canada. *Archives of General Psychiatry*, **50**, 947–951.

Masi, R. (1993) Multicultural health: principles and policies. In R. Masi, L. Mensah & K.A. McLeod (Eds) *Health and Cultures I: Policies, Professional Practice and Education*. London: Mosaic Press.

McAuliffe, E. & MacLachlan, M. (1994) No great expectations (V): Back to the future. Changes. *International Journal of Psychology and Psychotherapy*, **12**(3), 175–182.

McDonald-Scott, P., Machizawa, S. & Satoh, H. (1992) Diagnostic disclosure: a tale of two cultures. *Psychological Medicine*, **22**, 147–157.

McKinlay, J.B. & McKinlay, S.M. (1981) Medical measures and the decline of mortality. In P. Conrad and R. Kern (Eds) *The Sociology of Health and Illness*, New York: St Martins Press, pp. 12–30.

Mensah, L. (1993) Transcultural, cross-cultural and multicultural health perspectives in focus. In R. Masi, L. Mensah & K.A. McLeod (Eds), *Health and Cultures I: Policies, Professional Practice and Education*. London: Mosaic Press.

Moghaddam, F.M., Taylor, D.M. & Wright, S.C. (1993) *Social Psychology in Cross-Cultural Perspective*. London: Freeman.

Mrazek, P.J. & Haggerty, R.J. (Eds) (1994) *Reducing Risks for Mental Disorders: Frontiers for Preventive Intervention Research*. Washington, D.C.: National Academy Press.

Mumford, D.B., Nazir, M., Jilani, F. & Baig, I.Y. (1996) Stress and psychiatric disorder in the Hindu Kush: a community survey of mountain villages in Chitral, Pakistan. *British Journal of Psychiatry,* **168**, 299–307.

Mumford, D.B. Whitehouse, A.M. (1988) Increased prevalence of bulimia nervosa among Asian schoolgirls. *British Medical Journal,* **297**, 718.

Murdock, G.P. (1980) *Theories of Illness: A World Survey*. Pittsburgh: University of Pittsburgh Press.

Nakanishi, N., Tatara, K. & Fujiwara, H. (1996) Do preventive health services reduce eventual demand for medical care? *Social Science and Medicine,* **43**, 999–1005.

O'Conners, W.A. & Lubin, B. (Eds) (1984) *Ecological Approaches to Clinical and Community Psychology*. Malabar, Florida: Robert E. Krieger Publishing Company.

Oakley, P. (1989) *Community Involvement in Health Development: An examination of the critical issues*. Geneva: World Health Organization.

Ornstein, R. & Sobel, D. (1987) *The Healing Brain*. New York: Simon & Schuster.

Pedersen, P.B. & Ivey, A. (1993) *Culture-Centered Counselling and Interviewing Skills: A Practical Guide*. Westport: Praeger.

Poliakoff, M. (1993) Cancer and cultural attitudes. In R. Masi, L. Mensah & K.A. McLeod (Eds). *Health and Cultures I: Policies, Professional Practice and Education*. New York: Mosaic Press.

Prince, R. (1987) The brain-fag syndrome. In K. Peltzer & P.O. Ebigbo (Eds) *Clinical Psychology in Africa*. Enug, Nigeria: Working Group for African Psychology.

Proctor, R. (1988) *Racial Hygiene: Medicine under the Nazis*. London: Harvard University Press.

Ridley, A. (1994) *Making Sense of Illness: The Social Psychology of Health and Disease*. London: Sage.

Rogers, W. (1991) *Explaining Health and Illness: An Exploration of Diversity*. Hertfordshire: Harvester Wheatsheaf.

Rogler, L.H., Malgady, R.G., Costantino, G. & Blumenthal, R. (1987) What do culturally sensitive mental health services mean? The case of Hispanics. *American Psychologist*, **42**(6), 565–570.

Rushton, J.P. (1995) Construct validity, censorship, and the genetics of race. *American Psychologist*, **50**, 40–41.

Sachs, L. (1987) Evil Eye or Bacteria? Turkish migrant women and Swedish health care. Stockholm: University of Stockholm.

Sarson, S.B. (1974) *The Psychological Sense of Community: Prospects for a Community Psychology*. San Francisco: Jossey-Bass.

Sartorius, N. (1989) The World Health Organization's views on the prevention of mental disorders in developed and developing countries. In B. Cooper and T. Helgason (Eds) *Epidemiology and the Prevention of Mental Disorders*. London: Routledge.

Schumaker, J. (1996) Understanding psychopathology: lessons from the developing world. In S.C. Carr & J.F. Schumaker (Eds) *Psychology and the Developing World*. Westport, CT: Greenwood Publishing Group.

Schwarzer, R., Jerusalem, M. & Hahn, A. (1994) Unemployment, social support and health complaints: a longitudinal study of stress in East German refugees. *Journal of Community and Applied Social Psychology*, **4**, 31–45.

Shweder, R.A. (1991) *Thinking Through Cultures: Expeditions in Cultural Psychology*. Cambridge, Mass. Harvard University Press.

Simons, R.C. (1985) The resolution of the latah paradox. In R.C. Simons & C.C. Hughes (Eds) *The Culture Bound Syndromes: Folk Illnesses of Psychiatric and Anthropological Interest*. Dordrecht: D. Reidel, pp. 43–62.

Singer, M., Flores, C., Davison, L., Burke, G., Castillo, Z., Scanlon, K. & Rivera, M. (1990) SIDA: the economic, social, and cultural context of AIDS among Latinos. *Medical Anthropology Quarterly*, **4**, 72–114.

Smith, P. & Bond, M. (1993) *Social Psychology Across Cultures: Analysis and Perspectives*. London: Harvester Wheatsheaf.

Steptoe, A. (1991) The links between stress and illness. *Journal of Psychosomatic Research*, **35**, 633–644.

Steptoe, A. & Wardle, J. (Eds) (1994) *Psychosocial Processes and Health: A Reader*. Cambridge: Cambridge University Press.

Sue, S. (1994) Delivering mental health services. Paper presented at the International Congress of Applied Psychology, Madrid, 17–22 July.

Tajfel, H. (Ed.) (1978) *Differentiation between Social Groups: Studies in the Social Psychology of Intergroup Relations*. London: Academic Press.

Triandis, H.C.; Bontempo, R.; Villareal, M.J., Asai, M. & Lucca, N. (1988) Individualism and collectivism: cross-cultural perspectives on self in-group relationships. *Journal of Personality and Social Psychology*, **54**, 323–338.

Uchino, B.N., Cacioppo, J.T. & Kiecolt-Glaser, J.K. (1996) The relationship between social support and physiological processes: a review with emphasis on underlying mechanisms and implications for health. *Psychological Bulletin*, **119**, 488–531.

Varma, V.K. (1988) Culture, personality and psychotherapy. *International Journal of Social Psychiatry*, **34**, 142–149.

Vega, W.A. & Murphy, J. (1990) Projecto Bienestar: an example of a community based intervention. In *Culture and the Restructuring of Community Mental Health: Contributions in Psychology*. Series No.16. Westport, CT: Greenwood Press, pp. 103–122.

Vincent, C. & Furnham, A. (1996) Why do patients turn to complementary medicine? An empirical study. *British Journal of Clinical Psychology*, **35**, 37–48.

Vinck, J. (1994) The role of health psychology in the promotion of public health. Paper presented at the International Congress of Applied Psychology, Madrid, 17–22 July.

Weinman, J., Petrie, K.J., Moss, R. & Horne, R. (1996) The Illness Perception Questionnaire: a new method for assessing the cognitive representation of illness. *Psychology and Health*, **11**, 431–445.

Weiss, M.G.; Raguram, R. & Channabasavanna, S.M. (1995) Cultural dimensions of psychiatric diagnosis: a comparison of DSM-III-R and illness explanatory models in south India. *British Journal of Psychiatry*, **166**, 353–359.

Weisz, J.R., Suwanlert, S. Chaiyasit, W. & Walter, B.R. (1987) Over- and undercontrolled referral problems among children and adolescents from Thailand and the United States: The wat and wai of cultural differences. *Journal of Consulting and Clinical Psychology*, **55**, 719–726.

Westbrook, M., Legge, V. & Pennay, M. (1993) Attitudes towards disabilities in a multicultural society. *Social Science and Medicine*, **36**, 615–623.

Westbrook, M., Legge, V. & Pennay, M. (1994) Causal attributions for deafness in a multicultural society. *Psychology and Health*, **10**, 17–31.

Westermeyer, J. (1989) *Mental Health for Refugees and other Migrants: Social and Preventive Approaches*. Springfield, Illinois: Charles Thomas.

Winnett, R.A., King, A.C. & Altman, D.G. (1989) *Health Psychology and Public Health: An Integrative Approach*. New York: Pergamon Press.

World Health Organization (1948) *Constitution of the World Health Organization*. Geneva: WHO.

Wray, I. (1986) Buddhism and psychotherapy: a Buddhist perspective. In G. Claxton (Ed.) *Beyond Therapy: The Impact of Eastern Religions on Psychological Theory and Practice*. London: Wisdom Publications.

Wrenn, C.G. (1962) The culturally encapsulated counsellor. *Harvard Educational Review*, **32**, 444–449.

Zola, I. (1983) Oh where, oh where has ethnicity gone? In I. Zola (Ed.) *Sociomedical Inquiries*. Philadelphia: Temple University Press.

# INDEX

# Related titles of interest from Wiley...

## The Influence of Race and Racial Identity in Psychotherapy

### Toward a Racially Inclusive Model

**Robert T. Carter**

Describes the past and current understanding of race by mental health professionals. Racial identity is used to understand therapy process and outcome as reflected in a racially inclusive model of psychotherapy.

0-471-57111-3   320pp   1995   Hardback

## Black in White

### The Caribbean Child in the UK Home

**Jean Harris Hendriks and John Figueroa**

This thought-provoking book addresses sensitive issues affecting Carribean children growing up in the UK, drawing on the authors' experience of child psychiatry, adoption and fostering, education, welfare systems and the law.

0-471-97224-X   154pp   1995   Paperback

## Treating the Changing Family

### Handling Normative and Unusual Events

**Edited by Michele Harway**

Examines how non-normative events, non-traditional family constellations, and contemporary socio-cultural issues (violence, AIDS, ageing and ethnicity) impact on family development and functioning.

0-471-07905-7   384pp   1995   Hardback

## Counselling the Culturally Different

### Theory and Practice

### 2nd Edition

**Derald Wing Sue and David Sue**

"... considered a classic in the multicultural field."

**Journal of Multicultural Counseling and Development**

0-471-84269-9   336pp   1990   Hardback